T0272393

The Anatomy of Deception

The Anatomy
of Deception

Conspiracy Theories, Distrust, and
Public Health in America

SARA E. GORMAN

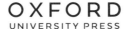
OXFORD
UNIVERSITY PRESS

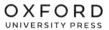

Oxford University Press is a department of the University of Oxford. It furthers
the University's objective of excellence in research, scholarship, and education
by publishing worldwide. Oxford is a registered trade mark of Oxford University
Press in the UK and certain other countries.

Published in the United States of America by Oxford University Press
198 Madison Avenue, New York, NY 10016, United States of America.

CIP data is on file at the Library of Congress
ISBN 978–0–19–767812–1

DOI: 10.1093/oso/9780197678121.001.0001

Printed by Sheridan Books, Inc., United States of America

For Robert, amor vincit omnia
and
For the courageous interviewees in this book who fearlessly
shared their stories about trust and distrust with me

Contents

Acknowledgments

Writing a book is at once an intellectual and emotional process, and it is never done alone. I would like to express my gratitude to all the wonderful people who helped me write this book. First, I thank all of the brilliant scholars and medical and public health practitioners, without whose contributions to the study of trust in health and science, misinformation, and health disparities, it would have been impossible to write this book. I am particularly grateful to the tireless efforts of so many physicians and public health professionals who work on a daily basis to restore trust in the healthcare system. I'd like to thank in particular the following scholars, who all generously served as interlocutors at some stage during the writing of this book: Céline Gounder, Heidi Tworek, Jan-Willem van Prooijen, Joseph Uscinski, and Kathleen Hall Jamieson. I am very grateful to the anonymous reviewer of the book whose input was critical in shaping and improving the final product. I am also very grateful to the wonderful people at Oxford University Press, including my fabulous editor, Sarah Humphreville, whose insight and input were always very much appreciated.

I would very much like to thank all of the members of my two organizations, Critica and Those Nerdy Girls, for always cheering me on and providing constant intellectual fodder for my ideas. Our work at Critica was very much front and center in the conceptualization of this book, and I would like to particularly thank David Scales, an exceptionally talented physician and scholar and a good friend. I am extremely grateful to the Robert Wood Johnson Foundation for providing funding for much of the work we do at Critica. I am also deeply grateful to the Board of Directors of Critica for ensuring that we can continue to do our work in a way that maximizes our impact.

Finally, there are many amazing people in my personal life who have provided endless support along this journey. I am deeply grateful to my sister, Rachel Moster, and my brother-in-law, David Moster. They have shown deep interest in my work on this book since day one, and I thank them for always inspiring me with their intellectual prowess and sustaining me with their warmth and encouragement.

This book was written with deep concern for the future of our country and the wellbeing of its inhabitants. This deep concern was made all the more pressing as I thought about all the American children who will have to bear the consequences of whatever world we create for them. There are three children in particular that occupy my mind: my niece and nephew, Jonah and Hannah Beth Moster, and my son, Raphael Kohen. I thank them all for their ceaseless light-heartedness during a time when I was constantly facing some very serious thoughts about our collective future. To Raphael, I say there are no words to thank you deeply enough for all the ways in which you have opened my mind and heart. You are an inspiration and a thorough joy.

There are three additional people who have collectively sustained me with their unending love and support. To my father, Jack Gorman, I think you have read every single word of text I have ever written since I learned to write. Your brilliance is an inspiration, and I am indebted to you for the intellectual gift you have given me. To my mother, Lauren Gorman, you are a genius psychiatrist with astounding insight into the life of the mind, which has definitively shaped the way I think about people and the world. I am eternally grateful to you for always showering me with warmth and love. Finally, to my husband, Robert Kohen, you give me everything I need to accomplish all the things that I could ever want. Words are inadequate to express my gratitude, but I thank you for being my rock and my muse.

Author's Note on the Interviews in This Book

As a way of providing more color around the concept of medical mistrust and conspiracy theories, I decided to conduct interviews as part of the work for this book. You will see descriptions and quotes from them interspersed throughout. It can be difficult to find firsthand accounts of medical mistrust and conspiracy theories, especially in this post-COVID moment. As a general rule, empathy has always been a large part of my approach to my research and writing on topics such as misinformation and science denial, and I wanted to be able to describe people's experiences in a way that was both accurate and demonstrative of the nuances of medical mistrust and belief in conspiracy theories. Drawing readers into individual stories felt like the best way to ensure that there could be a better understanding of why these attitudes arise to counteract the too-common automatic rejection of people who may hold these beliefs, which damages any attempt to build back trust.

The interviews in the book were mostly conducted between January and April of 2022. The questionnaire I used is published at the back of this book. All participants were asked the same questions, with follow-up questions in certain cases as appropriate. Most interviews lasted between 45 and 60 minutes. The interviews are separate from any work done by my nonprofit research organization Critica. I sought IRB review from an independent IRB (Salus IRB). Salus IRB determined that IRB approval for this work was unnecessary as it was not concerned to be contributing to generalizable knowledge and did not meet the criteria for Human Subjects research.

Participants were initially recruited via social media, with calls for participation going out on my personal Facebook, LinkedIn, and Twitter accounts. After that, the recruitment method was mostly snowball sampling, in which I asked interviewees to recommend other people I should interview. As detailed in the Introduction to this book, there was a wide range of ages, genders, geographic locations, occupations, education, and income levels among the interviewees. Interviewees were promised that names and other identifiable information would not be included in the book. I transcribed notes and specific quotes during the interviews on my personal device.

Introduction

In February 2023, I interviewed a woman who had spent upwards of 30 years in the pharmaceutical industry who, between tears, told me that she was afraid of what the COVID-19 vaccine was doing to people. Because she still works in the pharmaceutical industry, she asked me many times to be careful about what I shared about her. Yet in the same breath she wanted the "truth" to be known: that pharma companies knew the vaccines were dangerous and pushed them forward regardless. That same day, I spoke to a middle-aged retired steel mill worker with sarcoidosis. He was on disability and Medicaid and was a far cry from my previous caller's comfortable life in one of the wealthiest neighborhoods in the United States. And yet, his story was much the same. To say that mistrust in healthcare is common in the United States, particularly in the aftermath of the COVID-19 pandemic, is perhaps an understatement. When I recruited interviewees for this book by asking people to contact me if they distrusted medicine and healthcare, I was instantly overwhelmed with replies. It made my mission in this book that much more urgent and relevant.

This book examines how we got to this place of widespread mistrust in healthcare, health-related conspiracy theories, and the proliferation of misinformation about every health topic imaginable. But it also tends to the deeper structural issues that drive and exacerbate these problems. Over the course of the coming chapters, I draw a straight line between the structural problem of access to healthcare and the crisis of trust in local and federal health and public health institutions. Rather than treating lack of access as a public, social problem and mistrust as a private, psychological factor, I suggest that the two are actually closely aligned and the relationship between them is dynamic and bidirectional. Access drives trust, and trust also drives access. We need to stop asking the question: "What is wrong with people who can't trust the healthcare system?" and instead ask: "What is the healthcare system doing that is pushing so many people to distrust it?"

I also examine some of the major "macro" social problems in our country right now and suggest that their relationship with the crisis in healthcare is not actually that distant. The sense of isolation and abandonment that ensues from a recognition that the government cannot take care of its own citizens has led to a widespread feeling of disillusionment that has made authoritarian and populist viewpoints more attractive. I argue that the right to healthcare and a right to well-being are some of the most fundamental rights of any democracy, and the failure of the American healthcare system to protect its citizens has led to a widespread turning away from the very systems that underlie our country's democratic system. As a result, a turn to the far right, with a deepening of despair along the way (often referred to as "deaths of despair"), can be seen as a turn away from the systems of well-being that have failed so many people. I also conducted over 70 in-depth interviews with people who either expressed high levels of distrust of healthcare or who had a close family member who did. These interviews yielded many important insights, the most important of which is the idea that struggling to access quality healthcare leads to distrust in the medical enterprise full stop. In making this argument, I am by no means condoning acts of violence and hatred that happen on the far right. There is no excuse for any form of ideology that creates vicious in-groups and out-groups and proposes violence as a solution to societal problems. However, as we are living with the consequences of this widening ideology, I am trying to get to a place of understanding where some of the fuel for this fire is coming from. Perhaps in identifying this "fuel," we can also think about a road to reform of some of our social systems that would actually make a difference.

In this Introduction, I will give a short summary of these themes and then outline the arguments of each ensuing chapter. I will also summarize who was interviewed and some of the emergent patterns from this exercise.

Medical Mistrust: Definitions, Prevalence, and Equity Issues

Traditionally, medical mistrust has mostly been measured as a person's trust or distrust in their direct medical providers. Over the course of the pandemic, the average person's interaction with broader healthcare systems and public health institutions increased as a result of much more frequent and pervasive communication by organizations such as the Centers for Disease Control and Prevention (CDC) with the general public. One of the arguments of this book is that the notion of medical mistrust needs to be updated. It is no longer focused on attitudes toward providers, but includes a much broader sense of trust or distrust in institutions and the systems of health and public health that surround people.

The pandemic represented a serious blow to trust in healthcare and public institutions among both the general public and among clinicians themselves. Over the course of the pandemic, both patients and clinicians developed a greater degree of suspicion about recommendations coming from the government.[1] Some have noted that it can be difficult to build clinician-patient trust when even clinicians don't fully trust the recommendations and the healthcare institutions making them.[1] So in this case, we see a kind of intertwining of the twin challenges of trust in larger healthcare institutions and trust in individual clinicians. Between May and October 2020, trust in the CDC decreased, while trust in other government agencies (FEMA and USPS) increased, even despite recent scandals within the USPS.[2] There were substantial declines in trust in the CDC among those who wanted to vote for Trump in 2020 or who were not voting at all.[2] Trust in public health institutions and trust in science' had an important impact on the extent to which people took preventive behaviors during the pandemic, even regardless of political affiliation. For example, 80% of Republicans who trusted science in one survey reported feeling that social distancing was important versus 55% of Republicans who did not trust science.[3]

In 2021, the social science research center NORC at the University of Chicago did a very comprehensive survey of both patients' and clinicians' trust of different components of the healthcare system. Overall, they did find that patients had higher trust of personal clinicians than of any other component of the healthcare system, including the healthcare system as a whole (64% of patients said they trusted this), government agencies (56%), pharmaceutical companies (34%), and insurance companies (33%).[4] There were some interesting differences in the extent to which doctors and members of the general public trusted healthcare institutions. For examples, members of the general public say they trust hospitals at a higher rate (72%) than physicians do (60%).[4] There was also quite a disparity between the extent to which physicians think patients trusted them (98%) versus what percentage of the general population said they trust their personal physician (83%).[4] In general, people's trust in clinicians increases with age and income, but trust is lower among non-White individuals.[4]

There were also some important findings in this survey around the relationship between systemic and interpersonal trust and physicians' and the public's confidence in the general ability to change health behaviors and maintain adherence to treatment recommendations. There is a general belief in the field of medical mistrust that trust in individual clinicians is higher than trust in the healthcare system ("systemic" trust), which includes trust in governmental public health agencies that communicate with the public, such as the CDC, and that the two types of trust do not necessarily interact; that is, a person can have extremely low trust in the system but have a high level of trust in personal clinicians. The consequence of this has in some cases been that many people do not worry too much about low systemic trust because they think interpersonal trust (trust in an individual clinician) will be high enough to result in good treatment and health outcomes. This is wrong in a number of ways, not least of which is the fact that during a public health crisis like a pandemic, much of a person's behavior that will determine both individual and community health outcomes will be preventive and will not involve a personal clinician at all. But one of the other reasons this sentiment is misguided is that, as we see in this NORC survey, it probably isn't true that there's no relationship between systemic and interpersonal trust. For example, the NORC survey found that people with a high level of trust in the healthcare system are more likely to say that doctors trust what they say (87% versus 67%), that doctors spend sufficient time with them (80% versus 61%), and that doctors care about them (79% versus 52%).[4] This finding suggests that, contrary to prevailing opinion, it is in fact possible that lower levels of systemic trust may result in an erosion of confidence in a variety of interpersonal factors that may subsequently decrease people's trust in their clinicians as well. It is therefore extremely important that general trust in the healthcare and governmental public health systems be maintained.

There is another factor here, the concept of self-efficacy, which is the notion generally describing people's self-confidence in their ability to activate certain behavioral changes. Importantly, physicians tend to overestimate patients' ability to adhere to treatment plans, with 93% of them agreeing that most patients can adhere versus 81% of patients agreeing with this. In addition, 59% of clinicians believe that patients can make lifestyle changes, while only 49% of patients say the same.[4] As I will argue throughout this book, self-efficacy is not only an important driver of behavioral change, but also a component of trust in government health sources. People with high levels of confidence that they can understand and apply complex health and science information to their own lives generally feel less duped and controlled by government health and science communication. A better and more realistic understanding of patients' self-efficacy among clinicians would be a good place to start in building this skill in the general population.

What impact did the pandemic actually have on trust in the healthcare system among both clinicians and the general population? The NORC survey found that there were no major changes in trust in the healthcare system among patients and physicians as a result of the pandemic. For 53% of physicians and 56% of the public, trust levels stayed the same. However, there was still decreased trust among 30% of physicians and 32% of the public, which is not insignificant.[4] A fair number of physicians (43%) reported a decrease in their trust in government health agencies as a result of the pandemic.[4] On the one hand, many doctors previously believed their workplace was supportive. They believed their workplaces offered good access to care and reduced disease transmission. Yet only 75% of physicians thought their workplace supported their well-being during the pandemic.[4]

Perhaps not surprisingly, patients identified physicians as trusted partners during the rollout of the COVID-19 vaccine. Asian Americans reported higher levels of confidence in their doctors rolling out the COVID vaccine than other racial and ethnic groups.[4] Democrat respondents were 1.5 times more likely than Republicans to report confidence in their doctor to administer the COVID vaccine.[4] The impacts of COVID-19 on patient and physician trust remain to be fully identified. Yet it is fair to say that the contact that the average American had with the public health system and governmental institutions that plan for and run responses to disease threats increased during the pandemic. This exposure resulted in more reflection on trust in system-level actors in the healthcare system, which has become an increasingly important component of how people think and make decisions about individual health.

The trust literature importantly focuses a good deal of attention on how levels of trust, both systemic and individual, differ across racial and ethnic groups. As Bogart and colleagues have argued, mistrust has been conceptualized as a form of coping that fulfills epistemic (desire to understand), existential (desire to control), and social (desire to maintain a positive view of self or one's in-group) motivations under a state of uncertainty (such as COVID-19) and in the face of continued threat (such as discrimination).[5] In this formulation, mistrust can be seen as a response to a negative set of circumstances, such as the uncertainty caused by a pandemic or the everyday experience of discrimination faced by many people of color in the United States and elsewhere. It is, in this way, a coping mechanism. Learning not to trust authority figures and systems helps people shield themselves from the potential impacts of discrimination and exclusion. By shunning the system that oppresses them, people feel less beholden and less affected by subsequent discrimination and mistreatment. As a result, we might expect to see higher levels of mistrust among underserved and excluded populations. In this case, Bogart and colleagues' study looked at a convenience sample of Black Americans living with HIV. They assessed general COVID mistrust and associations between mistrust and COVID-19 treatment behaviors and future vaccine hesitancy attitudes and behavioral intentions. The study found that 97% of subjects endorsed at least one mistrust belief. The most prevalent mistrust belief had to do with the government withholding information about COVID-19. More than half of participants expressed hesitancy around future vaccination and treatment, and one-third said they would definitely not get vaccinated against or treated for COVID-19.[5] In general, only one-fifth of respondents said Black people could trust clinicians, although three-quarters noted that individual clinicians usually have their best interest in mind.[5] Bogart and colleagues also found lower levels of trust, higher rates of vaccine hesitancy, and reluctance to get treated among people with less education.[5]

The pandemic brutally exposed the extent of the disparities that exist in delivery and receipt of healthcare services in the United States. The idea that Black and Latinx Americans (especially Black Americans) distrust the healthcare system is ubiquitous throughout the literature on medical mistrust and has become a staple of most studies of vaccine hesitancy. The narrative usually goes that because Black people especially were subject to horrible mistreatment by the healthcare and public health systems in the past, the most egregious and infamous example being the Tuskegee Syphilis Study, they have in some ways compensated for the harsh realities of this history by refusing to trust the healthcare system or any individual within it. Of course, there are many problems with this account. For one thing, and as I will argue further in Chapter 2, most Black people do not think consistently about the Tuskegee Syphilis Study or any other awful experiment in American history as a way to make sense of their feelings of trust or distrust around clinicians and the healthcare system. There is an everyday experience of racism and discrimination that many Black and Latinx citizens experience that contributes strongly to feelings of distrust. Furthermore, the notion that hesitancy is based only on historically motivated distrust is not entirely true in these populations and places too much of the onus on victims to "get over it." While historical racism is clearly an important factor here, it must be understood in the context of continuing, contemporary forms of discrimination and racism that continue to sow distrust.

In addition, types of distrust are too often conflated across populations. Chapter 2 will study at length the differences in the types of distrust felt by predominantly Black and predominantly Latinx populations. The drivers and sequelae of these different types of distrust are not exactly the same and should not be discussed in the same breath. The idea that we can apply a one-size-fits-all solution to distrust across such varying populations is a mistake and can only fail.

There is another significant type of identity that intersects with medical mistrust that I have not mentioned yet but is probably at the forefront of many people's minds as they read this: political identity. While I am not a political scientist and cannot claim to analyze the current political situation with any kind of authority, given the unfolding of events especially over the past few years and the intense politicization of health issues such as the COVID-19 pandemic, I have found it necessary to comment on politics and political identity in various places throughout this book.

That disclaimer aside, it is important to recognize that the relationship between political partisanship and medical mistrust and associated correlates such as vaccine hesitancy is not always so straightforward. A clever study by Choi and Fox looked at relationships among public health institution trust, political partisanship (as measured by degree of trust in Donald Trump), and vaccine hesitancy. As the authors note, there are basically two hypotheses about how partisanship aligns with vaccine hesitancy. One is that there is something about partisanship per se that causes vaccine hesitancy. This is also known as the "exogenous" hypothesis. The other is that there are outside factors that correlate with partisanship, such as distrust in government, that are the true cause of higher rates of hesitancy among members of particular parties. Distrust in government and certain personality characteristics may be associated with both conservative party identification and vaccine hesitancy.[6]

In their study, Choi and Fox found that distrust in public health institutions (and by extension, the government) was a much greater predictor of vaccine hesitancy than partisanship as a concept. This is not entirely surprising, as many studies have shown the influence of distrust in government on vaccine hesitancy, even before the pandemic.[7-11] In this study, Choi and Fox found that distrust in public health institutions was indeed a much stronger predictor of vaccine hesitancy than either trust in Trump or self-proclaimed party membership. While it's true that when science is unclear, people tend to fall back on their political worldviews, the underlying level of distrust still played an important role in determining certain kinds of health behaviors. While people with low levels of trust in public health institutions claimed holding those views for a long time, even before the pandemic, there were still high levels of trust in personal clinicians in this group.[6]

In this study, among those who had low levels of trust in public health institutions, only 49% were vaccinated, regardless of their feelings about Trump specifically.[6] However, among those who had low trust in public health institutions, those who had high levels of trust in Trump had even lower rates of vaccination (41%) versus those who said they did not trust him (56%).[6] In this study, demographic factors had less of an impact on vaccine hesitancy than levels of trust in public health institutions, suggesting that in some cases we might be focusing on the wrong factors in the battle against vaccine hesitancy and refusal, at least in the case of COVID-19 vaccines. A large proportion of people who said they mistrusted public health institutions but trusted Trump had confidence in their personal physicians. A substantially lower number who distrusted both public health institutions and Trump had high levels of trust in their personal physicians.[6] Those who mistrust public health institutions reported having low levels of trust in local and national newspapers but had higher self-proclaimed trust in social media than those with higher levels of trust in public health institutions.[6] The likelihood of at least one vaccine dose among those who had trust in public health institutions and mistrust in Trump was 90% versus only 43% among those with low trust in public health institutions and high trust in Trump.[6]

What is the overall lesson here? To be certain, vaccine hesitancy refers to a complex conglomeration of attitudes and likely behaviors that cannot be attributed to one motivation or driver. However, it does seem to be the case that trust—specifically the more global, government-level trust in public health institutions—has an important role to play here. While many book-length projects have treated the issue of trust in health and medicine, the tendency has overwhelmingly been to focus almost exclusively on the clinician-patient relationship with particular attention to doctors. There has been some great literature written on the more systemic level of health-related mistrust in certain demographic groups, particularly among Black Americans, best encapsulated in Harriet Washington's seminal work

Medical Apartheid, to which I will be returning extensively in Chapter 2. But in this day and age, in the wake of COVID, a new level and threat of political violence and instability, and a right-wing media empire that sows the seeds of conspiracy theories in an alarmingly large number of American citizens, it felt like the right time to pursue a wide-ranging project that focuses not only on systemic mistrust in public health institutions, but also on the impact of the broader mistrust both in the government and in each other on Americans' desire and ability to seek out and procure quality healthcare. Throw in the backdrop of a population beleaguered with outrageous medical bills and poor access to even the most basic levels of medically necessary and preventive care and we have the perfect conditions to study the intertwining phenomena of access, trust, and conspiracy beliefs that now define not only our medical and healthcare system but, for many of us, our everyday lives.

The Twin Healthcare Crisis: Access and Mistrust

It is fairly well known by now that the United States ranks surprisingly low among developed nations for general health outcomes, coupled with exorbitantly high costs.[12] The COVID-19 pandemic also highlighted another major problem with the U.S. healthcare system: inequities and disparities in access and care. As of a survey done in 2021, 9.2% or 30 million Americans did not have health insurance;[13] 30.1% of Hispanic adults and 14.1% of non-Hispanic Black adults do not have health insurance, compared to 8.7% of non-Hispanic White people.[13]

While these statistics point to both a global issue of lack of good access to healthcare, particularly among Black and Hispanic adults in the United States, it does not tell the whole story of how lack of access drives all of the potentially dangerous attitudes and behaviors discussed in this book, from mistrust to conspiracy theories to vaccine hesitancy and lack of compliance with other public health safety measures. In preparation for writing this book, I interviewed dozens of people who were (or had relatives who were) highly distrustful of medicine and healthcare, or who held actual conspiracy beliefs about the healthcare system (or both, which did occur in many cases). These interviews, which I will pull from throughout the book, nudged me toward one resounding conclusion: it is poor access to healthcare that primarily drives mistrust. As people try but fail to get the healthcare they need, they often turn, in their abandonment, to alternative treatments and viewpoints. They become suspicious of a system that does not let them in.

The same thing can be said on a much wider scale about the government's abandonment of so many people by failing to provide an adequate social safety net, which includes universal access to quality healthcare. Feeling abandoned, many people turn toward alternative viewpoints, calling for alternative government orders, which can lead in some cases to despair and in others to political extremism, such as we see on the far right. It will be a mainstay of this book that the healthcare crisis is very much at the center of *all* of these phenomena and not just circumscribed to medical mistrust, because it represents such a widespread and palpable failure of government to care for its people. If a key element of a democratic society is to procure and ensure the well-being of the citizens within it, then democracy has failed in the United States, and the concomitant extremism and even political violence we now see on the rise are part and parcel of the same phenomenon, exemplified by an epic failure of our government to provide people with adequate healthcare, which in many cases leads to an inability to maintain a dignified existence. I wholeheartedly agree with Angus Deaton and Anne Case when they argue in their book *Deaths of Despair* that the failure of the healthcare system, not the economy per se, is actually at the center of the uptick in suicides and overdose deaths among a certain demographic of White males that we have seen in the past decade or so. In this book, I will be expanding upon this enlightening argument by showing that the access crisis, which was only exacerbated and highlighted by the pandemic, has led to a widespread feeling of unease and distrust that has ultimately turned many people away from the mainstream and toward an alternative way of thinking that can be very dangerous.

I am, of course, not the only one to make this argument. In the wake of the pandemic, some have noted that inequities, especially in access to COVID-19 vaccines, drive skepticism about the motives of vaccine makers.[14] Trust is indeed routinely undermined by financial burdens and poor access to healthcare. When care is unaffordable, patients don't trust that their well-being is at the center of the motivations of their healthcare providers and the healthcare system, and they start questioning motives more forcefully.[1] Historically, some have argued that high-deductible insurance plans specifically drove trust down. While these plans were supposed to empower patients, they often left them having to make big healthcare decisions without enough information, and in many instances kept them from seeking the care they needed due to fear about what would be owed under astronomical deductibles.[15] In an intriguing article and podcast series about "MMS," the "miracle mineral solution" that is basically bleach, Kristen Brown, a journalist for *Bloomberg*, tells the story of a woman named Anna, who one day started vomiting violently after ingesting this toxic concoction and recounted that she did not want to call an ambulance because it was too expensive.[16] Her lack of insurance was one of the factors that she thinks led her to miracle mineral solution in the first place. In her words: "If you're someone who doesn't have health insurance, it's a lot easier to just go online and buy something like MMS." As Brown further notes in the article, not having medical care contributes to distrust.

Several people have noted, with good reason, that we currently have a narrative around vaccine hesitancy that blames individuals, when we should really be thinking about the systems around them. By pointing to the fact that individual Black and Latinx Americans have high levels of mistrust in the healthcare system, we are ignoring the fact that there are major issues with their interactions with these systems, including poor access and discrimination.[17] Black communities in particular often have fewer providers to access and less access to care and medical services. Some of this unequal access to care is actually due to decades of disinvestment via racialized policies and practices, such as redlining and segregated cities.[17] Any account of vaccine hesitancy that does not take this context into account is misguided. Some of the policies early in the pandemic around vaccination may actually have inadvertently alienated Black Americans. In New York City, for example, there were rules around making vaccine appointments online and proving New York City residence. These rules may have been prohibitive to some Black residents of New York City.[17] These kinds of structural barriers may also reduce trust.

Some have argued that part of the hesitancy around COVID-19 testing and vaccination might have something to do with people's skepticism that these services would really be free.[18] In these cases, a combination of distrust in what officials were saying (that testing and vaccination would be free) and people's feelings about access (or lack thereof) collided to result in less-than-optimal health behaviors and, in many cases, bad health outcomes. We do know that people who experience good continuity of care and who have a higher volume of annual doctors' visits report higher rates of trust in both doctors and the healthcare system.[19] There is no question, then, that there is a strong relationship between access and trust in the United States.

This should not necessarily be surprising, as structural issues such as access greatly color people's feelings about the healthcare system and its operation in this country. Access to healthcare is indeed one of the great enduring problems in 21st-century America, and it should not come as a shock that this general failure on the part of our government to secure people's ability to live healthy lives would impact their feelings about not just the healthcare system, but also the broader government institutions that run and regulate it.

When trust gets really low, people are much more susceptible to believing false and even outlandish ideas. This is where another major theme of this book, conspiracy theories, comes into play.

Conspiracy Theories Go Mainstream

In a survey conducted in 2020 with a representative cross-section of the U.S. population, consumption of conservative news predicted an increased belief in conspiracy theories, and engagement with mainstream news predicted a decreased belief in conspiracy theories.[20] Further, conspiracy theory beliefs predicted levels of mask wearing and intentions to vaccinate during the height of the COVID-19 pandemic.[20] While exposure to COVID-19 misinformation has never been sufficient to "cause" belief in COVID-19 conspiracy theories on its own, there is a clear overlap between high levels of consumption of misinformation and belief in conspiracy theories.[21] There has been an ongoing debate about whether belief in conspiracy theories affects actual behaviors. Some have argued that they do, because there can sometimes be an observed direct effect of belief in conspiracy theories on compliance with government public health measures.[22] On the other hand, it is possible that what is observed as a direct effect is really indirect and mediated by trust.[22] That is, conspiracy theories are highly associated with distrust in government sources, and this distrust is probably the key factor that drives the lack of compliance. We may never know what the true answer is here, but it is clear that some combination of distrust and belief in conspiracy theories has a real impact on people's willingness to follow government public health measures. What is new, especially in the aftermath of COVID, is with what facility people now weave the narrative, more consciously recognizing that lack of access and other structural issues result in an erosion of trust at the point of care. Also novel here is the weaving together of several large cultural factors that all have a significant basis in healthcare system failures: medical mistrust, conspiracy theories, and an increasing level of political radicalization and rejection of government order.

Some level of belief in conspiracy theories appears to be relatively common in the population. In one study, respondents were presented with 22 different popular conspiracy theories, and only 9% did not believe in any of them.[23] Partisan conspiracy theories that blame the other political party for conspiring to create some bad outcome are pretty widely supported on both sides of the political aisle, with about 37% of Americans believing that Trump colluded with Russia to win the 2016 election, 28% believing that Hillary Clinton gave Russia nuclear materials, and 20% believing that Barack Obama faked his citizenship in order to become president.[23]

When it comes to COVID, about 29% of Americans believe the threat of COVID was exaggerated in order to hurt Trump's legacy as president, and 31% believe that the virus was created and spread on purpose. These COVID conspiracy beliefs are sort of in the "middle" of other conspiracy beliefs in terms of frequency of belief—they are less prevalent than ideas about the 1% controlling the government, but more prevalent than some of the more outrageous conspiracy theories that circulate in this country, including the idea that school shootings are "false flag" events.[23]

In an interesting study by communications experts Daniel Romer and Kathleen Hall Jamieson, participants were asked about their belief in three specific COVID-related conspiracy theories, including the belief that the pharmaceutical industry invented the virus for profit, that China created and spread the virus, and that the CDC purposely blew the pandemic out of proportion.[24] As might perhaps be expected based on the discussion above, there was an inverse relationship in this study between belief in conspiracy theories and undertaking methods to control the spread of the disease, as well as intention to vaccinate against it.[24] Romer and Jamieson also found that there was a higher rate of belief in these conspiracy theories among non-White participants.[24] Interestingly, this study also found that people who were "unsure" of these conspiracy beliefs were more likely to believe in conspiracy theories in general, but were also more likely to be persuaded out of these beliefs, so this represents an important population to focus on in efforts to combat misinformation and conspiracy theories.[24]

There are plenty of data to show a strong link between health behaviors and belief in conspiracy theories. Many recent studies have focused solely on preventive health behaviors relating to COVID-19, but there is an existing literature that suggests that engagement with *any* preventive health behaviors is lower among people who hold strong conspiracy beliefs. Belief in conspiracy theories has been shown to be associated with fewer annual exams, fewer visits to the dentist, and even lower rates of using sunscreen.[25] A 2020 study by Valerie Earnshaw and colleagues surveyed 845 people who were asked about belief in various COVID-19 conspiracy theories and questions about whom they trusted, including government sources, doctors, Anthony Fauci (former director of the National Institute of Allergy and Infectious Diseases and a chief medical advisor to former president Trump), and Trump. Participants were also asked about their vaccine intentions, since at the time the study was conducted in 2020 no vaccine was available for COVID-19 yet. They were also asked about how frequently they were following the hygiene and social distancing recommendations in place at the time. The study also importantly included a measure of medical mistrust.

In Earnshaw's study, one-third of participants reported believing in one or more conspiracy theories. In fact, those who did believe in conspiracy theories tended to believe in more than one.[25] A higher percentage of people who believed in conspiracy theories were younger, Black, and had a college degree, and they were also more likely to report higher levels of medical mistrust.[25] Participants with a high school education or less, who were male, White participants, and those with less knowledge about COVID-19 reported complying less frequently with public health measures such as social distancing and personal hygiene recommendations.[25] Participants who reported belief in conspiracy theories also had higher levels of mistrust of government bodies but, interestingly, also higher levels of trust in doctors.[25]

In addition to the debate about who believes in conspiracy theories and what kinds of behaviors and other beliefs these ideas lead to, there is an ongoing debate in American society right now about whether there has been an increase in conspiracy theory beliefs in the general population in recent years, especially as a consequence of the COVID-19 pandemic. On the one hand, there is political scientist Joseph Uscinski, who told me that, based on his research, there is no evidence that the rate of belief in conspiracy theories has gone up in recent years. Most others find this hard to grasp when conspiracy theories seem to have pervaded our information environment in a manner not really seen before, perhaps making it seem as though the whole country believes all of them.

I do believe Uscinski in his conviction here, but the question of the volume of belief in conspiracies in this country might be beside the point, at least for the purposes of this book. The purpose of my study of conspiracy theories in this book is to establish how the nature of these beliefs may have changed in recent years and, importantly, how they have been co-opted and manipulated by political and media personalities to make them easier to digest and incorporate into the everyday, general thinking of a much broader segment of the population. So while the belief in full-blown conspiracy theories might not be on the rise, the number of Americans who espouse some low-lying beliefs in something that sounds like a conspiracy theory, but may not have the full force of one, has most likely risen. The reason why this matters is because it has created an atmosphere in which the truth has become largely subjective and beside the point. In today's American culture, the "truth" is in the eye of the beholder and every conspiracy theory has become a "choose-your-own-adventure" tale in which the government is the enemy, the healthcare system is at the root of much of this evil, and the need to embrace a new line of thinking, whether it be some form of populism or far-right ideology, has become more urgent. And this brings me to the final major theme of this book that I want to highlight here before I give a preview of each chapter: the rise of the radical right and what this has to do with mistrust in the healthcare system.

The Rise of the Radical Right: Origins, Correlates, and the Healthcare System

Much like conspiracy theories, radical right ideology has become much more mainstream in the Republican Party over the past several years. These groups always existed, but were not generally accepted as a key component of Republican ideology.[26] This pattern is among the most troubling in American (and European) politics over the past several years. In some ways, radical right parties have accomplished this in part by focusing on a surge of migration (in both the United States and Europe) that has caused anxiety among many.[27] This kind of purposeful image reconstruction has served the far right well in mainstreaming their ideology. In the United States, some people certainly took advantage of Trump's presidency to spread right-wing extremist ideas, but the increased prevalence of this kind of ideology occurred well before the 2016 election.[28]

Far-right ideology is steeped in White supremacist ideas, but many far right-wing ideologies are equally focused on anti-federal government attitudes.[29] Not surprisingly, then, institutional distrust is a key component of the story of the rise of the radical right in the United States.[29] The rise in right-wing ideology and political violence we are experiencing in the United States at the moment is not necessarily a new phenomenon. The bedrock idea that White Christian men are somehow under threat from racial minorities and immigrants is not that different from the dynamic in the 19th century when partisan identity was conflated with race, ethnicity, religion, and immigrant status. At that point, many U.S. citizens felt they were losing ground to other social groups, and violence was committed not just by outliers but by regular individuals in the course of their normal daily activities. This is similar to what we are seeing now, with political violence or inclinations in that direction being committed by a more mainstream group of people.[30]

As the fringes become more mainstream, the actions of the far right have become harder to predict.[31] The online environment also makes it easier to cut off pieces of extremist ideology and disassemble and reassemble so it is closer to what one wants to believe. As will be discussed in Chapter 3 on conspiracy theories, the decentralized nature of extreme political ideology that appears on social media allows people to take these ideas and make them their own, rather than having to believe in a certain set of beliefs wholesale. This can allow less extreme individuals to start buying into more extreme ideologies.

Extreme right-wing ideology and populism often thrive on negative communication and rule-breaking, so there tends to be a focus on demanding radical solutions and blowing up the current structure.[32] As will be discussed at length throughout this book, this promise to "blow up" the current structure is appealing to a wide range of people who feel particularly abandoned by the government and the social safety net it is supposed to, but doesn't, provide. These feelings of abandonment have been preyed upon by certain groups on the right, including partisan ideological groups, the right-wing media, and even the right-wing political mainstream.

A major part of this break of the social contract has actually come from the healthcare system. Democracies hold the promise of looking out for citizens' well-being as a matter of definition. The fact that our society has not honored this promise cannot be without serious consequences. Angus Deaton and Anne Case have argued with considerable force that the phenomenon of deaths of despair, a particular set of deaths that have been on the rise over the past few decades due to suicide and drug overdose, often related to the opioid epidemic, in many ways has the failure of the healthcare system to thank.

Both the strain that our incredibly expensive and unsustainable health-care system has put on the economy and the sense that people are not being looked after by their government have led to an epidemic of despair. I believe something similar is going on with the rise of the radical right: people are not only experiencing economic strain that is caused in large measure by the burden of the healthcare system, but they have also become fed up with a system that does nothing to protect their livelihood. The system that is sup-posed to protect our health and well-being has instead become a breeding ground for extreme violence and tragic death.

In Their Own Words

As part of the original research for this book, I conducted upwards of 70 interviews with people who had high levels of mistrust in doctors and the healthcare system, or who had close family members who felt this way. Participants were recruited via ads on social media between May 2022 and February 2023. This was not a random sample and not representative of the entire U.S. population, and as a result, there may have been some bias in the sample. However, this was a high volume of in-depth interviews with a wide array of people from very different walks of life and is still instructive in our understanding of the current state of medical mistrust.

Among those who told me they felt they couldn't trust doctors or the healthcare system was a large contingent of people with chronic illnesses, in-cluding sarcoidosis, chronic Lyme, congenital heart defects, and other med-ical conditions, including hip dysplasia and interstitial cystitis. I interviewed people who were on disability and state-run healthcare, people who had seven-figure salaries at major U.S. corporations, and everything in between. Included in this sample were both U.S. citizens and people who immigrated from a variety of countries in Latin America, Southeast Asia, and the Middle East. There was a range of educational levels, from less than high school to advanced and doctoral degrees. Among those who spoke to me about family members with extreme views about medicine and healthcare, there was likewise a range of representation. The family members described by my interviewees again had a range of levels of education and came from a va-riety of countries, including Canada, Sri Lanka, and Norway, among others. There was a relatively balanced mixture of genders and ages, although most family members described tended to be people's parents, who were mostly middle-aged or older. A range of U.S. geographies was represented, including both urban and rural.

The results of these interviews will be interspersed throughout this book, but there are three main themes that I want to emphasize from the start: (1) medical mistrust can be deadly; (2) problems accessing the healthcare system feed distrust directly; and (3) the way the U.S. public health system managed the COVID-19 pandemic pushed some people with previously high levels of trust into strong feelings of distrust.

Let's look at a few examples. In February 2023, I received a panicked email from someone who said she saw my ad on Twitter and wanted to share that she had a blood pressure of 171/120, that she had gone to the emergency room, but that she had been mostly ignored, so she left. In her description of this incident, she also shared that she had "several congenital disorders" and she felt done with trying to prolong her life. She shared that she felt it took too much energy to get doctors' attention and that "no one really cares." I also had numerous other people tell me that they no longer went to the doctor because they were afraid or didn't see the point. Some of these people had a history of heart problems or diabetes or other chronic illnesses that require the regular care of physicians to avert serious complications. The sheer number of people who told me stories either about themselves or other people that indicated a straight line between distrust and mortality was striking.

The straight line between access and distrust was also striking in these interviews. One woman described her parents, who were immigrants from Pakistan, as having had relatively good access to healthcare in their native country due to living in a city and having universal healthcare. She shared that she believed a lot of her parents', and especially her mother's, distrust in the healthcare system arose when they moved to the United States and they had much poorer access to care. She thinks her mother relied on alternative treatments out of necessity and came to distrust mainstream medicine as a result. A wide range of other interviewees who had either themselves moved or had family members who moved from other countries with universal healthcare systems to the United States told me very similar stories about losing access and subsequently losing trust.

One interviewee told me she had been diagnosed with interstitial cystitis as a child and she never felt well until she was in her 40s. When I asked her about her access to healthcare, she shared that she had good access as a child, but as soon as she left her parents' house she was on her own and had to buy her own insurance. It was extremely expensive for her at the time and she struggled to make ends meet as a result. She admitted to having panic attacks every time she went to pick up her prescriptions because she became nervous about the cost. Ultimately, she told me: "I would rather kill myself than go through what I experienced before again. I am not doing that, PERIOD."

Then there are the innumerable stories about people who go bankrupt because they cannot afford their medical bills. This is surprisingly common in the United States. There was a poignant example of this among my interviewees, a woman with a chronic congenital hip condition. Growing up she had good health insurance, but lost it when she was in her 20s. She felt her public insurance was certainly sub-par, and she felt she experienced very different treatment from clinicians from this point on. Sadly, due to her condition, combined with pregnancy and childbirth and associated bills, she ended up selling her house and going bankrupt. Nervous about racking up bills, she and her husband stopped going to the doctor. Importantly here, she points to these financial problems arising from medical bills as the start of her questioning the trustworthiness of doctors and the healthcare system: "I did a lot more digging and learning about doctors, medical institutions, medical options and started questioning everything in most rigorous ways that I know had medical professionals frustrated with me. I can care less because my mistrust kept and still keeps eroding by the year."

A transitioning woman with severe mental health issues described the marriage of access and trust in a way that felt unacceptable and also unforgettable. She described the "nightmare of the healthcare system" as she tried to find services for anxiety, depression, and post-traumatic stress disorder (PTSD). At the time she was on disability and shared that it took her until she was 36, after many years of actively looking and searching, to finally have a social worker and a case manager assigned to her. She finally found about programs that were included with medical assistance that she thought she had needed for years and "could have vastly improved [her] life had [she] found out about them."

This same individual had some eloquent words to say around the cascading effects of poor healthcare access on the rest of society. As she shared, it is plausible to think that poor healthcare access could be having a marked effect on the economy:

> Many small studies the world over have shown that such things [e.g., increased access to healthcare] lower crime rates, improve working conditions which improves the workforce, which can in turn have a

cascading effect on many things. People who are healthy, happy, and able to support themselves are more likely to spend more in other areas of interest which ultimately means more money in the economy, and frankly even means more money going back into healthcare systems and research to continue to improve.

The idea that the poor functioning of the healthcare system has cascading effects, especially on the economy, is one that I will spend some time exploring in the pages to come.

It may come as no surprise that many people I interviewed identified the COVID-19 pandemic and the response to it as a key moment that either created or accelerated their distrust in the healthcare system. Some of these people had underlying feelings of distrust and suspicion, but some of them, interestingly, did not. When it came to what pushed people over the edge, a lot of it had to do with either the vaccine or advice they viewed as inconsistent from government sources. For many people, hesitancy about the vaccine or confusion about guidelines acted as gateways into more extreme, conspiratorial beliefs, usually involving intense suspicion of the government, the pharmaceutical industry, and doctors. One woman told me that she had generally been trusting of the healthcare industry and was a nurse herself, but she felt strongly that the government had forced people to take the COVID vaccine and that the concept of informed consent was dead. Another person told me that she had always been trusting of vaccines and was completely up to date on all shots before COVID, but she just felt that the COVID vaccine did not work and she was suspicious of how quickly it came out. Another interviewee who had worked in the pharmaceutical and biotech industries for over 30 years also told me she was always up to date on her vaccines before COVID, but developed suspicion around the COVID vaccines in part due to how quickly they were developed (in her view). She became convinced that the vaccines were in fact harming people, causing "turbo cancers," heart arrhythmias, and severe blood clots. She became so distressed that she even told me: "I have days where I just cry about what's happening. People are still rolling up their sleeves."

For others I interviewed, COVID was, as one person put it, "the nail in the coffin." For these individuals, there had always been a relatively palpable sense of distrust in the healthcare system, and the COVID-19 crisis and the response to it only pushed them over the edge. Many of the people who felt this way had bad experiences with prior treatments and surgeries or had chronic conditions or chronic pain that was unexplained or untreated. For this population, a burgeoning distrust of doctors became full-blown distrust in the entire healthcare enterprise by several years into the pandemic.

The Structure of This Book

The major themes of this book are surrounding the topics just discussed: medical mistrust, conspiracy theories, and the associated rise of the radical right in the United States. The book seeks to understand the unraveling of our democracy through the lens of the loss of institutional trust that has accompanied the collapse of our healthcare system. Each chapter will focus on one key area that tries to bring these topics together, culminating in a Conclusion that brings the whole picture together in one interpretation of the state of affairs and the future of our democracy and our healthcare system and the ways in which they are intertwined.

Chapter 1 outlines the traditional understanding of medical mistrust and argues that our current large-scale struggle with this phenomenon is in fact much more complex than the usual story. The chapter complicates the relationship between interpersonal and institutional mistrust when it comes to healthcare and trust in individual healthcare professionals and suggests that a better, more nuanced understanding of the real, modern nature of medical mistrust is essential in finding ways to combat it.

In Chapter 2, I extend the discussion of medical mistrust to examine the phenomenon of medical mistrust in Black and Latinx populations specifically. So much of the discussion of mistrust in these populations has traced everything back to medical malfeasance that occurred many decades ago. While past events such as the Tuskegee Syphilis Study have undoubtedly left an enduring mark on the ability especially of Black Americans to trust the healthcare system, focusing only on this example as the sole cause of the mistrust in these communities is unhelpful and nearsighted. In this chapter, I instead argue that everyday discrimination has more to do with medical mistrust in Black and Latinx populations than past events such as the Tuskegee Syphilis Study. In addition, I uncover why common efforts to group together the mistrust in different groups, such as Black and Latinx populations, is misleading and does not allow us to see the variegated, rich nature of medical mistrust in these different communities.

Chapter 3 takes on the question of the modern nature of conspiracy theories, with a focus on health-related conspiracies, but with some treatment of political conspiracy theories as well. Drawing from careful review of dozens of news clips from *Fox News* and interviews with conservative politicians such as Ted Cruz and Marjorie Taylor Greene, I make the argument that conspiracy theories in the modern age have become diluted, disassembled, and reassembled for common use. They appear in a more "casual" fashion in the everyday discourse of a wide array of mainstream politicians. These conspiracy theories are often what I call "decentralized," meaning they do not have a charismatic leader at the fore controlling all the messaging. As a result, it becomes easier for members of the general public to get pulled into ideas that may seem relatively innocuous but that really prove to be a gateway to a conspiratorial way of thinking. I argue that while the number of people proclaiming belief in full-blown conspiracy theories may not be higher now than it has been in the past, a form of low-level conspiratorial thinking has crept into more and more people's natural way of processing and making sense of the world.

A thorough understanding of the state of play of conspiracy theories brings the book naturally to an examination of the COVID-19 pandemic, in which we saw a major influx of new outlandish ideas about the mysterious virus. In Chapter 4, I focus on the governmental and public health system's response to the pandemic, with particular attention to the ways in which these actors communicated with members of the general public. I argue that the particular way in which failures of communication took place in response to the pandemic is actually a symptom of a failing democracy. Communication that sows mistrust in public health authorities and the health system in the midst of a health crisis shows signs of a democratic society in decline. I also discuss certain characteristics of the American political and healthcare systems that predisposed this country to having a poor response to the pandemic. Throughout the chapter, I discuss various ways in which this communication could be improved during a future health crisis, but this process will only work if our nation's democratic institutions, and citizens' trust in them, are improved.

Chapter 5 examines loss of trust in a variety of institutions and asks the question of whether lack of trust in the healthcare system is of a piece with this trend or is somehow unique. In this chapter, I argue that losses of trust in government institutions and in healthcare systems and institutions in particular are not unique phenomena, but all part of the same story. This chapter digs deeper into the idea that Americans feel abandoned by the social safety net and have in some cases become radicalized as a result of this failure. I also do a deeper dive into the different types of trust, how they are formulated, how they disintegrate, and start to pave the way for suggestions about how to rebuild it, which is very much the subject of the sixth and final chapter.

The book's final chapter takes a look at ways of remedying some of these problems. While the problems discussed throughout the book are vast and many of them structural in nature, I argue in Chapter 6 that there are ways to mitigate some of the issues we are currently seeing around mistrust, misinformation, and the spread of conspiracy theories. I argue that the breakdown of the information environment is both a cause and a result of the larger loss of trust and spread of conspiracy theories that have taken hold of both the healthcare system as well as other parts of American society in recent decades. While actually "fixing" the problems discussed throughout the book around conspiracy theories and institutional mistrust will require large, systemic changes to our government and corporate structures, it is still the case that in the interim, there are smaller solutions that can make a difference and change the course of ever-widening mistrust. In the end, while much of American society, with healthcare at the center, probably needs a makeover, it is still possible to see a silver lining in the gargantuan efforts of many researchers and practitioners who are trying every day to mitigate the impacts of conspiracy theories and mistrust in the healthcare system and beyond.

One thing that has often concerned me is that discussions about the problems with misinformation, distrust, and conspiracy theories are just that: focused on the problems and the problems alone. The scholarship and public discussions can become quite depressing as a result. While I spend considerable time in this book outlining the origins of these problems and diagnosing a series of serious problems with our healthcare institutions, I hope that there is enough material suggesting some solutions that this book does not leave people without hope. There is no question that we are living in an incredibly difficult time, with a lack of overall trust in our institutions, a disordered information environment, and a veritable crisis about what is in fact the "truth." It is also the case that many of these problems are not entirely new and that the more we can understand them, the better positioned we are to do something about them.

Systemic and structural problems with our healthcare system might be daunting, but it is far from impossible to make progress here. In the meantime, there is a lot that individual citizens can do to encourage others to seek out healthier information environments and check themselves when their frustrations with the healthcare system make them prone to taking up false and even conspiratorial ideas. There is no way to discuss these problems purely on the individual level, so of course some of the problems and their solutions will be large and systemic. This is going to require a kind of political will that may be difficult to see in the current environment. Nonetheless, we cannot shy away from the true heart of these issues just because solving them is difficult. Our democracy, our livelihoods, and our very lives depend on it.

1

"Above All, I Trust My Doctor"

Trust, Distrust, and Medical Decision-Making

It seems like a simple question: Whom do you trust for information on health? Most people have somewhat of an immediate answer to this question, usually involving some combination of family members, healthcare providers, friends, and the Internet. But this issue of trust in healthcare, from the macro level of the system all the way down to the individual provider standing before you, has never been more complex in U.S. history than it is today.

There is no question that overall, the U.S. population's trust in the healthcare industry writ large has been declining steadily for decades and is now at a particularly low point. In 1966, more than 75% of Americans reported having great confidence in the country's medical leaders. As of 2016, this number was down to 39%.[1,2] This steep decline is both alarming and curious, immediately begging questions about what exactly over the past few decades has resulted in such a sharp decline. This distrust extends outside of healthcare to general distrust of the federal government: in recent years, only 14% of the general U.S. public has reported believing that the federal government does the right thing most of the time.[3]

We need look no further than the COVID-19 pandemic to see a true crisis of trust in action. Conspiracy theories and vicious political fights accompanied almost every piece of guidance from the major federal health authorities, including the CDC and the Food and Drug Administration (FDA). Dr. Anthony Fauci, who was at one point the top infectious disease specialist in the country, was regularly stalked and received death threats from people who thought he was lying, suppressing information, or otherwise misleading the public. A series of events that seemed like they should be in no way political—a relentless virus that required relatively standard public health measures to contain—suddenly became the source of violent battles among people with differing values and politics across the country. People complained that the government changed positions on various topics, such as whether to wear a mask, too many times to be trusted, and they posited that pharmaceutical companies were burying evidence about the harmfulness of the vaccines. In their most extreme forms, conspiracy theories arose claiming that the vaccines contained microchips to allow government and private businesses to track citizens' movements and actions and that the virus was purposely created and released from a Chinese lab as a bioweapon. These conspiracy theories require that people believe that the government willfully withheld information from the American public, which is of course a hallmark of any conspiracy theory. Some have posited that conspiracy theories and distrust of the government and the healthcare system are major contributors to COVID-19 vaccine hesitancy, which accounts for the fact that our vaccination rate is just over 50% when it should be closer to 90% in order to achieve herd immunity and be able to move on from this pandemic.[4-6]

Despite this evidence for a trust crisis in the modern American healthcare system, it is actually far too simplistic to claim that Americans categorically and unilaterally distrust the system and disregard the health advice of government agencies and providers on a regular basis. The picture is in fact far more complex than that. Research conducted by my research organization Critica has, for example, found that people tend to trust their healthcare providers, even when they simultaneously harbor distrust of the healthcare system and the government.[7] Therefore, we are currently experiencing a major paradox when it comes to trust in the healthcare system: while trust in the system, comprising mostly the government structures that deal with health and medicine but also the pharmaceutical and insurance industries, seems to be at an all-time low, trust in personal physicians and other healthcare providers is actually quite high. Even so, most people cannot fully trust their doctors either, because they are always painfully aware of the (distrusted) systems surrounding these practitioners. This duality of simultaneous trust and distrust leads to an extended decision-making process in which people are not satisfied to consider only the advice of their personal healthcare providers, but are constantly gathering information from a wide array of sources, many of which can be misleading. The health and medical decision-making process thus becomes protracted, confusing, and dangerously open to a range of biases, the most insidious of which is often identity politics. But herein also lies an opportunity to improve the situation. If we understand that most people are not making instantaneous decisions based on faulty information or deeply rooted biases, but are instead deeply ambivalent, then there are many opportunities to intervene and improve the decision-making process. In this chapter, I will examine the characteristics and some of the underlying drivers of distrust in the healthcare system and demonstrate that, above all, Americans are ambivalent when it comes to trust of healthcare providers in particular. I will show that medical decision-making in such an ambivalent population not only makes people vulnerable to misinformation, but also allows for an opening to intervene and steer them toward the most evidence-based decisions. The end of this chapter will provide a practical description of just how to do this.

This narrative of ambivalence runs counter to the traditional narrative we have seen both in popular media and in the academic literature in the past several years. Declarations of a public trust crisis in healthcare have only increased during the pandemic and especially in the face of substantial amounts of COVID-19 vaccine hesitancy. Some have declared this medical mistrust phenomenon "the biggest health crisis facing the United States today."[8] Others have tied mistrust in the government overall to mistrust in the healthcare system, which is declining steadily and posing grave threats to our well-being.[9] A 2021 article in *Newsweek* declared that "American society is in the throes of a terrible and increasing crisis of trust" and that expertise will soon be of "limited utility" as a result.[10] All of these statements are in fact true. We are facing a major threat to our health and well-being as a result of generally dwindling trust in the healthcare system. However, I believe these examinations of the issue gloss over places where that trust still exists in quite a powerful way and eliminates any understanding of the high levels of ambiguous emotion Americans have about medicine and healthcare providers. Even as trust is dwindling, people are still wondering whether there is a way to continue to trust their doctors, and they are trying to reconcile continued trust in some elements of the healthcare system with flat-out distrust in others. If we are to start posing solutions to this problem of trust, it is essential that we ensure that we understand it better first.

A good example comes from an interview I did in early 2023. A woman who was unvaccinated and had been in the intensive care unit (ICU) for severe COVID became distrustful of the hospital system due to perceived incompetence and of her own primary healthcare provider due to what she viewed as constant questioning about why she was not vaccinated. She claimed not to trust her doctor anymore, but then admitted that she was still under his care and following his directions. When I questioned her on this, she backtracked and expressed feelings of ambivalence about her doctor.

Rather than flat-out distrust, COVID had for her, as for many others, shaken the foundations of her trust, but she was still not ready to let go entirely.

Before going further, let's make clear that there are many good reasons to mistrust the American healthcare system. Nor is the point of this chapter, and this entire book, to argue that people should simply be quiet and trust everything their doctors say. This could not be further from the truth. In fact, Americans have a myriad of completely legitimate reasons to absolutely distrust the healthcare system. The American healthcare system is notoriously and perhaps in some ways irreparably broken, with out-of-control costs, limited access, and poorer outcomes than any other high-income country. It is absolutely the case that the pharmaceutical industry engages in highly suspect and sometimes illegal behaviors in order to make a profit, and the ongoing opioid crisis is only one example of flat-out criminal activity by this industry. Physicians are often mired in conflicts of interest, financial and otherwise, that have been shown time and again to very much influence their decisions. We are over-tested, over-diagnosed, and over-charged. Every day, women across the country die of childbirth complications that are completely avoidable and uncommon outside of the United States. And the list goes on. Based on all of this, it is completely understandable that people would be wary of the healthcare system and of individual providers as well. However, very often people take this distrust in the overarching system to mean they should distrust the scientific basis on which legitimate health and medical recommendations rest. This is a mistake and can indeed have tragic consequences. In this book, I am not trying to argue that people should be taught to unequivocally trust their doctors and the larger system. I am, however, arguing that people should learn not to have all their interactions and decision-making be colored by broader, overarching distrust that is in many ways completely legitimate.

It is also important to understand how the pandemic affected trust in medicine and individual providers. While overall trust in personal physicians remains high, a substantial minority of people lost faith in their doctors when the pandemic laid bare a larger crisis in the healthcare system. People began to see individual providers and the system surrounding them and as they lost faith in the system, they started to question their providers too. Their ability to see these aspects separately, as most did in the past, somewhat collapsed. These consequences were very evident in nearly everyone I interviewed, but one example sticks out from a woman who expressed deep distrust of the entire healthcare system, from individual providers all the way to the CDC:

Obviously some measure of trust and cooperation is important with your family physician and your local health dept. If you need medication for pink eye say or you develop cellulitis, etc. etc. you have to be able to get a prescription and have a primary doctor to go to or if you need a water sample or soil sample you need a public health dept but more and more I think everyone is realizing how very very easily healthcare is influenced and in fact, manipulated and even owned by powerful pharmacology companies. The internet has made so much information available to us and as long as it is not censored then people can make up their own mind which is a good thing. Because as soon as you have some outside entity censoring information it takes away your own individual autonomy to make your own choices for your own body.

In this case, the interviewee is somewhat measured, while also acknowledging that the almost blind faith people had in their doctors before the pandemic will be difficult to revive. Another interviewee expressed concern that doctors were censored by the CDC, a thought she told me she had never entertained before the pandemic:

My distrust has grown over the years. Doctors are no longer allowed by the feds to provide needed medical care or address patients' concerns. I have lost very capable doctors for this very reason. There are very few physicians who will address a patient's concerns and explain medical results in detail. Too often I get passed off to specialists. I want a doctor who will treat me. Since COVID, I can no longer trust their expertise. It's limited to the CDC, WHO, and their affiliated hospital boards. I know my physical problems. I'm never listened to and given any credence. My healthcare is jeopardized since I don't feel I can address problems with my physician. Government needs to get out of healthcare.

In this case, this person felt very uncomfortable with what she saw as an intimate intertwining of government activity and the practice of individual physicians, specifically as a result of COVID. When I asked her more directly how COVID impacted her view of healthcare and doctors, she said: "COVID made me realize how overwhelmed doctors are and how much at the mercy of insurance companies doctors are when it comes to care. It also made me realize how vulnerable the United States healthcare system is to collapsing in on itself. If the pandemic were any more severe I had grave concerns there would be no healthcare system in the United States." In other words, before COVID perhaps there were issues with the healthcare system but one could at least trust one's doctor. After COVID, it became more difficult for people to separate their concerns about the healthcare system and the government running it from the individual clinicians who treated them. In this way, interpersonal trust (and distrust) *became* a matter of institutional trust (and distrust).

"I Don't Trust the Federal Government": The Crisis of Systemic Distrust in Modern Healthcare

Several surveys over the course of 2021 showed that Americans generally believed that the government was not to be trusted when it came to obtaining reliable information about the COVID-19 pandemic. About a quarter of Americans reported believing that the mainstream media were lying to them about COVID-19 and that there was some truth to the idea that the outbreak was at least partially planned by a malicious actor.[11] While it is true that the pandemic represents extreme circumstances that may not always mimic everyday life, it is also true that the crisis laid bare certain attitudes about organized medicine and healthcare that were already brewing, to say the least. Among these attitudes was a blanket distrust of federal (and sometimes state and local) health authorities who were providing vital information and guidance about this serious health threat.

Americans' distrust in the government and especially in healthcare should not be entirely surprising. The conspiracy theory discourse had already changed over the course of the 20th century from viewing aliens and other supernatural beings as primary threats to instead believing that the government itself was the conspirator.[12(pp19-20)] Medical conspiracies have been common for some time now, even before the pandemic. In general, 49% of Americans believe in at least one medical conspiracy and 18% believe in more than one.[12(p123)] A 2014 study found that 37% of Americans believe the FDA is deliberately suppressing natural cures for cancer because of drug company pressure.[12(p122)] These medical conspiracy theories run the gamut of topics and include notions such as that fluoride causes cancer and other serious health issues but is still being placed in water sources by public officials who are suppressing this information, and that the childhood measles-mumps-rubella (MMR) vaccine causes autism but that the government, particularly the CDC, is once again suppressing this information and continuing to give shots to children as part of a joint ploy with the pharmaceutical industry.

To some, these notions might sound "out there," particularly the idea that there is a coordinated effort to suppress scientific information by various government agencies comprising thousands upon thousands of scientists. While it is true that belief in the most extreme conspiracy theories is not terribly common, the discourse around organized medicine and health-care in this country is littered with paranoid thinking styles and conspiratorial beliefs. These "low-level" conspiratorial thought patterns form the basis of a common way of thinking about healthcare in this country: that the large institutions that oversee health and medicine are corrupt, but that individuals such as personal physicians and other healthcare providers *may* be trustworthy. Untangling these two beliefs from each other proves very difficult for a wide variety of Americans who often become confused and indecisive when trying to make important healthcare decisions. I will get to attitudes toward personal healthcare providers later in this chapter, but let's take a look at how these low-level conspiratorial thoughts about healthcare manifest in real time.

In his book on conspiracy theories, philosopher Quassim Cassam argues that conspiracy theories often serve an important purpose in society of forcing us to consider possibilities that we should entertain. Of course, more often than not, these ideas are too extreme to be adopted wholesale. But sometimes they open up conversations about fundamental issues of trust and incentives that do need to be addressed. For participants in focus groups and in-depth interviews conducted over the course of 2021 by me and several colleagues, it was certainly the case that low-level conspiratorial thinking was helping them work through real and often legitimate concerns they had about COVID-19 vaccines, vaccines more generally, and the general operation of the entire medical and healthcare systems.

For this series of studies, we interviewed 94 individuals in three disparate U.S. locations—Chicago, Newark, NJ, and central Texas—in January 2021. We selected these locations because they represent a diversity not only of geography but also of demographics and political views. In July 2021, we also interviewed a group of 30 African Americans and a group of 30 Latinx participants who self-identified as hesitant about the COVID-19 vaccine. We wanted to understand how experiences of systemic racism in medicine might impact people's decision-making around new medical technologies and the role that trust (or lack of trust) plays in their perception of the medical and healthcare systems. Subjects participated in online bulletin boards, in which they responded asynchronously to questions about trust, vaccine hesitancy, and other related topics. Subjects have 3 days to respond to all questions and cannot see the responses of others until they respond first. This brand-new information provides much-needed depth and explanatory power to general trends of uncertainty and ambivalence we can see in the published literature.

In his study of conspiracy theories, Cassam notes that their content matters less than people's vague sense that something is not right, usually with the government specifically.[13(p108)] Our study showed that low-level conspiratorial thinking is very common in the health and medical context, but that there was a lot of vagueness and many internal inconsistencies in these ideas. For example, in response to a question about whether the COVID-19 vaccine should be mandated, one participant in Chicago said: "I am not a conspiracy theorist but when the government starts mandating what you should do to your own body it seems sort of communistic." This participant is thinking broadly about what it means for the government to mandate something without specifically addressing the issue at hand. This kind of vagueness was rampant, as were frequently juxtaposed ideas that were contradictory. As one participant in Texas shared: "This is a sensitive question. As mentioned in the previous answer, if it is safe and effective, then it will benefit everyone, so everyone should be vaccinated. However, the government always abuses the power, so they may go beyond simply helping people beat the virus." This person is clearly uncertain—on the one hand, it may be important to at least nudge everyone toward getting the vaccine if it proves to be so safe and effective that it is essential. On the other hand, if the government "always" abuses power, how can she feel comfortable with that same institutional body issuing and executing a medical mandate? As we will see, this kind of conflicted, sometimes self-negating conspiratorial thought pattern is very common when it comes to managing doubts about healthcare and medicine. Thus we must also understand that rather than being faced with rabid anti-vaxxers, most doctors are faced with something potentially much more challenging at times: a person suffering from doubt.

Distrust in government-run medical and public health institutions has a few different underlying beliefs: the notion that anything government-run is inherently political and thus has ulterior motives that are not in the best interest of the public's health; that excessive equivocation and disagreement on the part of government health officials means they cannot be taken at their word; and the classic conspiracy belief that the government is willfully hiding seminal information from the public that may change their decision-making processes about vaccines and other health issues. There are also beliefs that the healthcare system has become too impersonal, that profits are leading the way to an inappropriate degree, and that technology has caused changes to occur too quickly.[14] Some people don't apply these ideas to every decision or health-related issue. For example, one participant in Newark talked about trusting "older" vaccines, but not newer ones because they have been "politicized" and "carry a lot of political baggage." One participant, also from Newark, said that she wouldn't trust the COVID vaccine if it came recommended by anyone with any political ties whatsoever: "Perhaps after a few years, if actual scientists (not talking heads) with no political ties at all do a study with no ulterior motives, social or political, and declare it to be safe, not based on opinions from 'experts,' which mean nothing, but based on actual data gathering which is open to the public to cross-examine and question." It is difficult, and probably impossible, to imagine a world in which there is zero government involvement in the development and manufacturing of a vaccine that needs to reach the entire U.S. population.

The notion that health officials' equivocation or changing their minds makes them less reliable or trustworthy is particularly interesting (and also troubling). One might expect that health officials being open about changing their minds might indicate a level of transparency that would make people trust them more. Instead, these twists and turns simply sow more doubt in the minds of those who are perhaps already unsure. We have heard this refrain frequently during the pandemic, with many people citing Dr. Fauci's change of heart about masks as a prime example of his utter untrustworthiness. How can we trust someone who cannot even get something seemingly so simple right the first time?

Participants in our study expanded upon this theme in abundance. One participant from Texas shared: "I do not read any information from big medical establishments anymore. The statements seem to change constantly and appear to have ulterior motives." Perhaps implicit in this statement is the notion that the changing statements are actually a sign or symptom of corrupt practices or ulterior motives. The assumption is that if no vested interests were involved, public health officials would be able to state the facts and stick to the facts. But because they are mired in an array of scandals and untoward alliances, as this narrative goes, they frequently change their position to appease whomever is necessary to maintain their personal interests. A participant in the Latinx study shared that "they have never kept their story clear and just because you are in government does not mean that you are completely sincere, we will never really know the truth and they simply keep changing their words. For example, with masks they say wear a mask, then they say you should wear it and then they say it's unnecessary, only it's always changing." Here, the underlying assumption is that there is some greater "truth" out there but that the government is suppressing it, resulting in conflicting information coming from government figures who apparently cannot "get their stories straight." There is inherent distrust of any new information that adds to or, worse, conflicts with previous recommendations or data. As one participant from the African American study noted, "I also am concerned about the news release of a Booster shot. Sometimes I wonder about the safety since the Booster was not mentioned initially." Just the fact that boosters were not mentioned initially but became a recommendation later is enough to make this person doubt the validity and honesty of the whole concept of the vaccine.

This phenomenon of changing views from updated data and information causing serious distrust is a big problem, especially during a fast-paced, ever-changing information environment such as a pandemic. Of course, science more generally is characterized by frequent change and updated viewpoints due to its empirical nature of inquiry, and medical science is no exception to this. While scientific data may change slowly and gradually over time in most cases, during a pandemic, dealing with a previously unknown disease with all attention turned toward studying it, it is not surprising that information and recommendations were being altered almost continuously. This created a very difficult information environment for public health officials to communicate with the general public, and it is clear from our research and the research of others that public health officials did not do a great job of addressing the distrust that would arise from changes in recommendations. Now that we can establish that changing recommendations are a key component of distrust and even the formulation of conspiratorial thought patterns, we can begin to pay more attention to how we communicate these changes.

Despite the high prevalence of conspiratorial thought patterns and notions about the government suppressing information and generally being corrupted by ulterior motives, we can detect a certain amount of ambivalence in many of the statements of distrust we see among members of the general public. This can be further substantiated by frequent survey findings that although Americans say they distrust the government, they also often report that they want the government to be more involved in solving the nation's problems.[15] Many people in our study voiced conspiratorial thoughts while simultaneously declaring outright that they do in fact mostly trust the medical establishment, and going back and forth between the two over the course of a single statement. As one participant in Texas put it:

> Well, I wouldn't doubt what the medical industry might say on a given topic just because I think I know more. But, I'm always curious if other professional fields, academia, or areas of the world agree with them. Again, because the medical industry is pretty freakin biased. And prone to creating and then denying problems (like the shit response to the AIDS epidemic or creating the entire opioid crisis).

This statement is wholly conflicted, at once admitting that the medical establishment has credible expertise (which is why he says he would not doubt them based on a faulty belief that he knows more) while simultaneously espousing conspiratorial thought patterns about ulterior motives and information suppression ("denying problems").

Another participant in Texas shared: "I typically have faith in what I see from the 'medical establishment' but unfortunately in our country research is funded by interested parties and that does not always coincide with what is best for everyone but rather what is best for those interested parties. Sometimes you must go a little further to know if the recommendation is genuine or not." Again, the elements of trust (or in this case, "faith") and the elements of serious distrust (e.g., believing that medical researchers have ulterior motives because of funding structures and that the establishment does not have the best interests of the public at heart) completely coexist in this statement. This simultaneous trust and distrust, this deep ambivalence about whether to believe what the medical establishment says, is even more pronounced in the highly fraught physician-patient relationship.

"I Trust the Advice of My Doctors": Trust and Distrust of Personal Physicians and Other Healthcare Providers

Even during the height of the pandemic, a Pew poll found that the majority of Americans reported trusting their doctors. In this study, 74% of Americans reported having a mostly positive view of doctors, and 57% believed that their doctor had their best interest at heart most or all of the time, with an additional 33% responding "some of the time."[16] The vast majority of participants in our study also said they thought their doctors had their best interest at heart. At the same time, the seeds of doubt could be seen even in this mostly positive survey. Only 15% of Americans felt that doctors are transparent about conflicts of interest most or all of the time, and only 12% thought doctors appropriately admitted mistakes and took responsibility for their actions.

This keen awareness of the coexistence of potentially trustworthy doctors inside an untrustworthy system seems to be troubling for many people who appear conflicted about whether or not to wholeheartedly embrace their doctor's advice. Statements in our study were full of contradictions, such as this one from the Texas group: "I trust doctors, researchers, scientists, the medical community if they don't have an agenda or don't appear to be politicized." Or this one, also from Texas: "Not sure. Lately because of so much wishy-washy statements that always seem to change I have grown in distrust towards large health organizations. But I usually trust local doctors regularly." When asked whom they trust most on medical and health matters, one participant in Texas said: "Generally speaking, my doctor. But, the American medical industry is biased and espouses some beliefs/practices that aren't true. So, I take it with a grain of salt (with things like obesity or maternity care, not vaccines)." All of these statements indicate a propensity toward trusting one's doctor, along with a shadow of doubt owing to wariness of the larger seemingly corrupt system in which doctors exist.

Participants were particularly concerned about the potential for doctors to be corrupted by pharmaceutical companies. As one participant in Texas put it: "Yes I trust them for the most part. Sometimes I think they are trying to push a certain brand of drug because they always prescribe it but usually they have pretty sound judgment." Although it doesn't appear here explicitly, this statement implies a concern that doctors may have financial conflicts of interest that cause them to over-prescribe the products of particular pharmaceutical companies. Even with this possibility, this participant does report trusting doctors, so the threat of ulterior motives related to potential pharmaceutical company corruption is not a "deal breaker." Another participant in the African American group said: "I find his advice convincing. The only thing I question is certain medications that he may promote, I would wonder if these were meds that he really thought would work or were they meds that he was getting perks to push." This statement is more explicit about the concerns surrounding financial ulterior motives stemming from the pharmaceutical companies, but once again this person still reports primarily following the doctor's advice. These types of double-edged statements, simultaneously declaring trust and undermining that trust with speculations about faulty incentives, were frequent in our study. This kind of simultaneous trust and distrust is also readily on view in other studies, such as a 2019 Pew poll that found that people trust their doctors, but also think they are not transparent about conflicts of interest or mistakes and errors.[17] More Americans now, as compared to 15 years ago, believe that doctors are interested in working for the public good, but more also think that doctors are at least partially in it for the profit, compared to the opinion of Americans 15 years ago.[18]

Even when participants reported a high level of trust of their doctors, there was still a pervasive desire to feel like decisions were made independently and that advice was personalized to their particular situation. This desire for personalization and independence is borne out by the literature as well, with one recent survey finding that around 75% of Americans wish their healthcare experiences were more personalized.[19] One participant in the African American group, in response to a question about whom they trusted for medical information, shared: "My doctor and the CDC. I trust the majority of what my doctor says. I trust the CDC also, but I feel my doctor personally knows me and how my body may react." This suggests some degree of skepticism about the CDC's advice simply because it is not tailored to this person's body and particular health status, whereas the doctor's advice can be personalized and thus more reliable. In the Latinx group, two participants talked about always questioning what is advised or prescribed: "When it comes to information about the body, I trust the advice of my doctors, but I always question what I was prescribed." Another participant, in response to a question about trusting the doctor's advice, said: "Yes I trust but always analyze my own decisions." These are qualified statements of trust, in which participants report that they do feel what might be described as a warm feeling toward their doctors, believing that their doctor is there to help them and guide them appropriately, and yet at the same time there is an inkling of a lack of complete trust, a sense that the doctor does not truly know them, and that they have to take matters into their own hands. Pair this with the fact that, as discussed above, people seem painfully aware of a large distrusted system surrounding even the most trusted of doctors, and we have a very complex situation. In the next section, we will see how this dual, simultaneous trust and distrust lead to a troublingly complicated approach to medical decision-making.

Trust, Distrust, and Medical Decision-Making

A study conducted in 2020–2021 by NORC at the University of Chicago found that even doctors have a lot of questions about the trustworthiness of the healthcare system as a whole. The percentage of doctors who say they somewhat or completely trust the healthcare system is not too much over half, and at 63% almost exactly matches the response to the same question from the general public, at 64%. This study also showed people's capacity to separate out different components of the healthcare system, some of which garnered drastically more trust than others. While 84% of respondents said they trusted doctors and 85% said they trusted nurses, only 34% trusted pharmaceutical companies and 33% trusted insurance companies.[20]

It seems eminently fair to say that it is not only possible but perhaps even common for people to trust doctors while completely distrusting the system to which they belong. However, it is not so cut and dry, as we have seen—people often find themselves questioning their doctors even as they claim to trust them wholeheartedly. So what effect does this confusion have on medical decision-making? How do people process and understand the information around them when their sense of trust and allegiance is so uprooted and sometimes even unpredictable, depending on the details of the issue at hand?

In this context, the decision-making process becomes complex, multi-layered, and nonlinear. People report gathering information and opinions from a wide variety of sources and people, and then it is not always clear how they actually utilize this information. For example, 1 in 4 Americans reports regularly using mobile apps for self-diagnosis, and about 45% of Americans report using a phone or tablet to manage and make decisions about their health.[21] There is also a strong bias toward any information that is about personal experience, prompting researchers to suggest that clinicians directly integrate narrative into their communications with patients.[22,23] In our study, we asked relatively open-ended questions about how people search for medical information online, how they decide what to trust and not trust, and how they combine this self-driven research with the advice of real people in their lives, including but not limited to personal physicians.

We found that while doctors almost always make the list of people that most go to for medical advice,[24] it is much more common for people to just start Googling and see where they end up. At least one-third of Americans use Google to find out more about actual or suspected health conditions.[25] Few people have a dedicated medical site they visit, such as WebMD, but are rather more prone to follow whatever Google might happen to bring up, whether it is accurate or not. Some combination of Googling, talking to a doctor, and consulting with family and friends was generally fairly common, as in this example from the Chicago group: "I Google a lot and ask my PCP and friends who work in the medical field who know a lot about the vaccines. I don't always trust everything Google says but I do trust my PCP and friends because they never gave me a reason not to and are usually right when it comes to my health concerns."

Part of the reason people seek advice from sources other than their personal physicians has to do with their overall distrust of the system surrounding their doctors. There is this sense that their doctor is generally knowledgeable and trustworthy, but that because there are potentially competing and some-times nefarious interests, it is vital to do one's own investigations.[26] Some are therefore automatically skeptical of doctors' motives, unless they have been able to vet their connections to industry:

I mostly decide based on who is hosting this person to speak. If he or she is being hosted by CNN or FOX or any mainstream media outlet, then au-tomatically it's NOT an expert and automatically should NOT be trusted. Anything the mainstream media says, I'm trained to believe the exact op-posite. If it's a doctor speaking in a medical context, preferably to other doctors and without any hint of a political or social agenda, then I'm more inclined to trust him or her.

This person trusts the input of doctors, but this trust is highly qualified. They must be speaking with absolutely no social or political ties apparent that could be influencing what they think.

This concern about ulterior motives extends to trust of individual public health officials, such as Dr. Fauci:

Fauci, while being the public face of much of the research to find a cure for the corona virus, is again, just a man. He makes mistakes like the rest of us, and isn't all knowing. So, as with any source of information or data, it is important to look up sources, discovered who sponsored the funding for the research, what their overall end goals are that are stated on their mission statement of their website, and cross check with multiple authorities on the same topic.

Here, we see an individual taking in what seems like a great deal of data and information in order to avoid being pulled in by someone's faulty incentives.

In addition to being skeptical of physicians and public health officials because of their potential ulterior motives, people overwhelmingly express a preference for information that is personalized to them or that is based on the personal experiences of others. Many express that looking into personal experiences and thinking about their own particular situation as part of their decision-making process allow them to take matters into their own hands and essentially exert more control over the situation. The suggestion here is that just listening to the objective advice of doctors is insufficient because it lacks a personal touch. By doing all this, people are signaling that their ultimate trust is in themselves and that they will feel most comfortable and satisfied with decisions they perceive as coming from them rather than being imposed by someone else. This is why people are generally uncomfortable with the concept of "choice architecture"—they want to continue to believe that they are making their own decisions.[27,28] Health decisions are no different, even if there is a fair amount of technical information involved that not every individual may fully understand.

One member of the African American group reported turning to the "self" for true knowledge about particular health topics:

> I normally turn to self research for health concerns. Ie [sic] internet, you-tube, etc. I find that although the doctors and physicians are knowledgeable, we are all human and they too can get it wrong. So with that I don't put my health concerns in hands of one source. Like to get opinions of people actually experiencing these things themselves not just dr's or specialist diagnosing someone with something.

Relying on self-research rather than the advice of doctors allows this person to gain control over the situation. Another participant in the same group suggested that her body is her ultimate barometer and what she trusts the most:

I trust the medical experts who I believe are honest and forthcoming, but mostly I trust me and my body, my body always lets me know when it is functioning at its best and when its [*sic*] not I am and will always be an advocate for my health, however I am not crazy if a Dr. tells me I have something or I have to do something I take it for what it is, but I will research to see what it is to get a better understanding and I will research to see if there is a holistic way to combat it if necessary before pumping loads of pills or shots, I also trust my friends and family especially if they have already experienced something that I haven't or know of someone who has and their information sounds valid (although I will still research for myself) but I trust they will give me the best information they have at the time.

Here the ultimate arbiters of the truth are this person's body and the self-research completed to better understand the issue.

Another individual actually ties all this back to memories of making poor decisions when guided by a doctor and better decisions when guided by a relative or a friend: "I trust people who have experience with dealing with certain conditions that are similar to mine because they have hands-on experience with managing a certain condition. I use my own judgment to determine if their advice is absolutely bonkers. There are times where I have received AWFUL advice from a medical doctor, but amazing advice from a non-medical friend or family member." Again, there is a premium on this notion of "hands-on experience" as opposed to simply what seems like abstract medical knowledge. This focus on one's own decision-making role in healthcare should not be terribly surprising in light of what has been called the "age of patient autonomy."[29,30]

In terms of actual decision-making, a number of participants talked about trusting their "gut" in the end: "I absorb information from various entities and go with my own 'gut' instinct to decide. I believe in the power of my foundation." Similarly, another individual shared: "I consider all sides and go with my gut after reviewing all the facts and data points. Ultimately, I am the sole responsible party for my health so it's important I do what's right for my own body." Perhaps difficult decisions are more easily made when there's a sense that you arrived at your own conclusions. There is also a strong inclination to feel like you were not taken in by some trick or overly persuasive tactics, as one participant in Chicago put it, in discussing the COVID vaccine: "I'm sure I heard positive things from government agencies on the news or on the web. It's good to hear but it still doesn't hold much sway to make me get it as my own personal experience has more of an impact. I'm not a sheep." This person is admitting to putting aside potentially sound advice from experts in the federal government in order to avoid feeling like someone else has in some way decided for her. In other words, in order to avoid feeling like a "sheep," it's important to decide to judge things for oneself, even if that involves disagreeing with known authorities on the topic.

This sentiment could be viewed in action when people were asked about intentions to get the COVID-19 vaccine and what factors might persuade them to do so. Not surprisingly, most people reported hearing a lot of advice on this topic from medical and public health officials but still wanted to feel as if they were making their own decision. Even when members of their family were vaccinated, people reported that this fact was not always influencing them to get vaccinated themselves: "Yes I know both friends and family members that have been vaccinated. It hasn't really change [sic] my timeline on pursuing vaccine. Once I've made up in my mind that I'm ready then that's when I will go ahead. I've always been raised to be a leader not a follower. So I don't do something just because someone else is doing it." This desire to be a "leader" rather than a "follower" seems prevalent in the decision-making process about important medical and health concerns, including the COVID vaccine. Others were similarly insistent on their independence of mind: "Yes as I stated previously 2 of my sisters were vaccinated. 1 fully 1 partially. 1 of my friends were vaccinated without issue. Most of my family and friends are not going to be vaccinated. Their personal decision doesn't affect my thinking or decision not to be vaccinated." One participant even pointed to an ability to resist persuasive information on social media as well as conspiracy theories: "I really don't believe in conspiracy theories, I try to be objective with the information I hear. I don't let myself be influenced." As we probably all know, it is difficult to imagine a situation in which anyone makes a decision that is devoid of influence. And yet, many people seem to be actively convincing themselves that they are free of persuasion when making health and medical decisions.

Why does this process of decision-making, in which people simultaneously trust their doctors and distrust the healthcare system and attempt to make their "own" decisions, matter so much? In part because it complicates a narrative we have been telling about science denial and misinformed medical decision-making for several years now. Much of the focus in this field has been on so-called "fast" thinking—automatic processes involving strong biases that negate the ability to sift carefully through data and facts. The idea is that people mostly use motivated reasoning, the process of interpreting information based on what one wants to be true, to understand the information around them.[31–34] There's also an assumption that people who doubt scientific and medical findings always engage in a kind of black-or-white inflexible thinking with no capacity to see the nuances involved in scientific findings.[35] What we have found recently, however, is quite the contrary. People are actually very conflicted when it comes to trust in doctors and the healthcare system, and this conflict results in a kind of slow, sometimes confused and confusing, medical decision-making process. This thought process may open them up to error in some ways but is in no way akin to the kind of automatic thought process involved in something like motivated reasoning. There are in fact many shades of gray in their thinking. If we can come to recognize that people are engaging in a thought process that is littered with contradictory ideas, then we can focus on drawing this ambivalence out in ways that will help them think more clearly and deliberately about scientific facts, rather than ultimately defaulting to a position of distrust that may not be appropriate in every situation.

Intervening in the Decision-Making Process

Many of the participants in our study and in many of the other studies cited here may be said to be showing signs of "science skepticism." "Science skepticism" has been an important concept of late due to its connection to adherence to COVID-19 containment guidelines (such as mask-wearing, vaccination, and social distancing). Scholars define "science skepticism" as a general lack of trust in science writ large. The extent of people's skepticism is generally socially derived. People intuit the extent of overall societal trust in science by observing informal social interactions, things they see in the media, and things they hear politicians say. They listen to how scientific topics, especially novel findings and new concepts, are discussed in order to basically guess the level of trust in science in the population at large at that moment in time. They then form a sense of their own trust in science largely based on this perception.[36]

Science skepticism goes hand in hand with another concept, often referred to as "anti-intellectualism." People with a high proclivity toward anti-intellectualism are also often high on the science skepticism scale. Anti-intellectualism has been specifically linked to inappropriately diminished concern regarding COVID-19, perceptions of relevant COVID-related risk factors and an often skewed perception of low risk, and lower willingness to engage with and seek out information from experts.[37] Anti-intellectualism, which can be conceptualized as general mistrust of experts and expert opinion, has actually been more predictive of rejection of COVID-19 science and containment measures than political affiliation.[38] In the case of vaccines in particular, the need for trust in multiple intersecting government institutions is profound. Vaccine confidence consists of trust in the legitimacy of political institutions that propose and provide the legal and regulatory frameworks for mass vaccination, in the healthcare systems and workers that deliver vaccines on the ground, and in the science that underpins vaccine efficacy and safety.[36] So trust on multiple levels turns out to be of paramount importance in the venture to improve vaccine acceptance.

This research suggests that trust is the linchpin of an effective response to any major health crisis. This trust is also absolutely necessary for the proper functioning of the healthcare system and to maximize the health of the general public. As we have seen, the so-called crisis of trust in health and medicine in the United States today is far from simple. Instead it is characterized by intersecting feelings of simultaneous trust and distrust and a desire to feel autonomous and in control of an increasingly technically complicated arena. Given these complexities and the abundant amount of ambivalence that thus enters into the medical decision-making process for most people, we actually have an opening to help increase trust in science and fend off science skepticism. But how do we do this?

We still do not have quite enough research on what kinds of interventions work to fend off skepticism about science and increase trust in authoritative health and medical institutions, especially when these deliberations are occurring online. Yet there are some suggestions both from the literature and from other, somewhat comparable scenarios and situations that can help us formulate some ideas. In a creative paper looking at methods of developing and maintaining trust in public health systems during food safety crises and scandals, the authors suggest that the tenets of public trust in these types of official organizations are: transparency; development of protocols and procedures; credibility; proactivity; putting the public first; collaborating with stakeholders; consistency; education of stakeholders and the public; building your reputation; and keeping your promises.[39] Some of these items may seem obvious and relatively self-explanatory. But a few require further thought and explanation. Even transparency, which seems like a must-have on a list of items that contribute to public trust, is not merely defined as sharing information as it comes up in an open and honest way. In fact, if that is all public institutions did during crises, people would be very unhappy and possibly suspicious. Part of the reason is because scientific information often emerges in a relatively slow, drawn-out manner, and during a crisis people want to be updated multiple times a day. Silence can even generate as much suspicion and distrust as providing false or not completely verified information. Public health institutions need to have a clear plan for how to continue communicating with the public during times when they actually *don't* have any new information. Can they anticipate how people will respond to differing scenarios based on what new information eventually reveals? Can they get in front of any objections, misinformation, or areas of serious distrust that could arise once new evidence comes into play? If they do not know exactly when new information will become available, they need to have a plan for how they will communicate that uncertainty, knowing that people may be particularly anxious and want answers.

"Credibility" is another area that may seem straightforward but is actually somewhat complicated. During a crisis, the public wants to hear from non-government-affiliated experts and to be reassured that these experts, even when deployed to share their opinions by the government, are able to maintain their impartiality. The suspicion of government spokespeople and actors was a major theme in our series of studies, and it is not surprising that this arises in the literature as a primary component of public trust during a crisis. But what degree of separation from potential "conflicts of interest" do these experts need to have? Since it is virtually impossible for someone to be completely devoid of external influences, how do we ensure that people have enough independence to be viewed as "credible" by most members of the general public? A 2011 report from the National Academies of Science suggests that the absence of conflicts of interest is one of the main components of trust in clinical guidelines.[40] This report sets an extremely high bar for conflicts of interest, basically asserting that individuals should divest themselves of all potential financial conflicts, including personal investments in companies that could potentially be deemed as influential in some way. It is difficult to know what level of absence of conflicts is needed to reassure people that government and non-government experts are credible. It most likely depends on the population and the particular issue or crisis at hand, but it is something that needs to be more closely examined to ensure that those who are called upon during a crisis are going to be trusted and believed by members of the public.

Obviously, these problems are not specific to health and should be seen in the larger context of declining confidence in the government overall. What is perhaps more important than just the declining confidence itself is Americans' perceptions of overall trust in the government. In a 2019 Pew survey, an overwhelming 75% of people reported believing that overall trust in the government was declining among Americans.[41] In general, people believed this flagging of trust had mostly to do with government issues around poor performance and, once again, conflicts of interest, specifically those involving money. Overall, people recognized that this lack of trust was a problem—64% reported believing that low trust in the government makes it harder to solve the country's problems. Important here is the *perception* of a trust issue in the American public. While trust may be low, especially in the midst of the COVID-19 crisis, perceptions can drive thoughts and behaviors that are based on false notions. For example, teenagers report thinking their peers drink alcohol at much higher levels than they actually do, and this can actually drive higher alcohol consumption in general in this population.[42] It is possible that people's trust in the government may be flagging in part because they perceive that everyone else's trust is flagging. So if this is not actually true to the extent that Americans think it is, it is essential to get more accurate information to people. The same is true of trust in medicine and the healthcare system—perception of generally low levels of trust can in turn drive those levels even lower.

To the extent that people's sometimes diminishing trust in their doctors and the healthcare system leads them to seek out information for themselves, usually online, it is important to understand what to do when people encounter misinformation in this venture. There have now been a number of studies looking at how to stop the spread of misinformation online, where the majority of people are exposed to it now. Some have suggested that priming people with an injunction to think specifically about accuracy makes them less likely to share questionable headlines on social media.[43] There is also the concept of "prebunking" or "inoculation." Just as a vaccine inoculates against a potential future encounter with a pathogen, "inoculation" in the context of misinformation means warning people about the potential for false information before they are exposed to it.[44-46] The common social media company technique of flagging information as "disputed" is effective, but only very modestly so.[47-49] Researchers have also found that closed-mindedness and limited reasoning capacity are more associated with the decision to share misinformation than is politically motivated reasoning.[50-53] Encouraging

someone to think more creatively or even just simply to think more rigor-
ously about what they are being asked to believe can help get them out of the
"closed-down" mindset that might be contributing to their belief in and willingness to propagate misinformation.

When faced with one-on-one conversations with someone who is
displaying distrust and science skepticism but with a high dose of ambivalence, how should a person, whether a private citizen or a physician, respond to encourage an increase in trust in scientific expertise? There are a
couple of principles of how to approach these situations that might make
the interaction more successful. Keep in mind, of course, that it might
take more than one interaction to make a difference in someone's thinking
and behavioral intentions. Note that these are suggestions for mostly one-
on-one interventions between any two people or between doctor and patient. There would likely need to be structural changes made to the medical
system to allow doctors the training and time to be able to carry out these
conversations. To that end, a broader consideration of needed structural
changes to the healthcare and medical system, both for the sake of these
types of conversations as well as more generally to build trust in the face
of issues such as conflicts of interest, will be included in Chapter 6 and the
Conclusion.

Draw Out the Ambivalence (Rather Than Shying Away From It)

It might be more accurate to say that Americans feel generally ambivalent
about their doctors and even the healthcare system as a whole than to say
they either trust or distrust them. There were elements of simultaneous trust
and distrust throughout our research and those of others, and confusion
about whether to believe the claims of personal physicians as well as of organized health-related government entities. This ambivalence may seem like
a problem, but it actually makes it easier in some ways to engage people in
open dialogue about trust in science, medicine, and the healthcare industry.

In this situation, it may be best to emphasize and draw out the ambivalence
as part of a technique based on a concept called motivational interviewing.
Motivational interviewing was first developed as a treatment for substance
abuse, which leans heavily on the idea that people mired in alcoholism,
drug addictions, or other addictive behaviors are actually ambivalent about

their addiction.[54] While they feel compelled to continue the behavior, they often have many negative feelings about how those addictions make them feel and what they make them do. As a result, they are always seeking a way out to some extent, but often fall short when the exit route is too difficult. Motivational interviewing positions the therapist to draw out this ambivalence and help the patient articulate deeper goals that are usually incompatible with the consequences of addiction. In the process of better articulating and recognizing ambivalence, patients are moved closer to a state of readiness to change. Motivational interviewing has been shown to be highly effective and has been applied to a broad range of other situations, including vaccine hesitancy.[55,56]

In the case of trust in doctors and the healthcare system, it will be especially helpful to get people to recognize that they are even ambivalent in the first place, as many may not realize this. Get them to articulate the fact that they do (and want to) trust their doctors but that they are very aware of the potential corruption in the system that surrounds him or her. Getting people to more carefully examine their distrust and realize that it may be causing them more difficulty making important decisions will help them approach the concept more carefully the next time they try to work their way through a complex medical issue. Recognizing the role that distrust is playing in their decision-making is a first step toward getting people to approach these decisions with a more critical eye.

Emphasize Self-Efficacy and Help People Further Their Own Research and Inquiry Skills

The concept of self-efficacy, observed and developed by psychologist Albert Bandura, refers to a person's belief in his or her ability to execute certain behaviors and reach certain goals.[57] It is a seminal element in behavior change, as it provides the motivation necessary for people to expend effort on sometimes arduous tasks to reach a goal. Self-efficacy has been discussed extensively in the health context, usually in reference to behavior changes around health issues such as weight loss, smoking cessation, and participation in preventive behaviors such as mammograms and colonoscopies. When people believe they have the ability to attain goals related to these behaviors, such as actually losing weight, they are usually able to mobilize the necessary resources to take action.

In recent years, there has been an active movement of "patient empower-ment" to ensure that patients can feel more included in healthcare decisions. The passion surrounding this movement suggests that it is common for people to feel disempowered when it comes to healthcare decision-making. It was clear from our research that people never want to feel as though someone else is entirely in charge of their decisions, no matter how much they trust them. So they take matters into their own hands, sometimes by trusting mis-information they see online or faulty ideas from friends and family members. This situation necessitates finding a way to build on people's sense of self-efficacy and independence surrounding healthcare decisions while also keeping them as close to professional and expert opinions as possible.

Although it may take some extra time, potentially requiring somewhat of a restructuring of our insurance reimbursement policies, doctors do have an important role to play here. Doctors can create a structured environment within which people can be encouraged to explore medical information on their own. This might involve getting a sense of where people normally look for medical advice and giving pointers based on accurate sources on-line. Doctors' practices can also provide general information about what to look for when judging whether a piece of medical information is accurate or not. In general, most doctors do not discuss the kind of independent re-search patients tend to do on their own time. If it does come up, it seems that doctors can sometimes be dismissive or not want to discuss it. This is a big mistake. The more doctors can encourage this kind of behavior in a way that is accurate and safe, the more patients will feel empowered by the doctor in their decision-making. In other words, doctors should embrace people's natural tendency to want to do some of this research on their own, and in-stead of insisting that only their word should hold sway, should actually teach people how to do this research effectively so they ultimately come to a medi-cally accurate decision.

Address Legitimate Reasons for Distrust

At the beginning of this chapter, I laid out some of the reasons why distrust in our healthcare system is completely warranted. These reasons were cer-tainly not lost on participants in our study. Among the reasons people in our study listed for being suspicious of doctors and organized medicine, there were a number that were completely legitimate and not stemming from misinformed conspiracy theories by any means. Several participants in the African American group discussed both historical examples of abuse of Black people, often by government medical and public health agencies, as well as deeply entrenched racism and general disregard within the health-care system. This topic will be covered in a great deal more detail in the next chapter, but in the meantime it is important to note that these grievances are completely understandable and are based on the reality of ongoing poor treatment of ethnic and racial minorities by our country's medical establishment.

A number of participants also mentioned legitimate reasons to be wary of pharmaceutical companies, including the very real fact that these companies are sometimes too influential with the FDA as well as with individual physicians. One participant mentioned the opioid epidemic, which is diffi-cult to put aside when dealing with public trust in the healthcare system. In very recent memory, the pharmaceutical industry did actually conspire to contain information about the harmfulness of a class of drugs in order to maximize profits. The result is at least 100,000 Americans dead in the period between the spring of 2020 and the spring of 2021 alone.[58]

This focus on actual breaches of confidence by key institutions in our healthcare system has to be addressed more directly. It should change our approach to rebuilding trust from an attitude of "why *shouldn't* people trust it?" to "why *should* people trust it?" It may be more helpful to examine with people what will happen if they trust an institution that does something untrustworthy versus what might happen if they fail to trust an institution that should have garnered their trust. What are the respective benefits and risks in these cases? Help people open up to the possibility that they might find some actions of the healthcare system to be questionable while still abiding by some of its recommendations. Most importantly, people should be allowed to voice these concerns without immediately facing a rebuttal. As has hopefully been abundantly established, it is possible for people to have doubts and still trust large portions of the system at the same time.

Stimulate Scientific Curiosity

Multiple studies have now confirmed the idea that science curiosity may be more influential than actual knowledge in determining how accepting people are of scientific facts and how easily they can shed biases and identity politics that make them more vulnerable to misinformation. One 2017 study by Dan Kahan, a professor of law and psychology, and colleagues had some surprising findings about science curiosity and political information processing.[59] This study found that politically motivated reasoning, a way of thinking entirely motivated by ideology and political identity, can be nearly fully negated by scientific curiosity, defined as motivation to seek out and consume scientific information for personal pleasure. It is important to note that science curiosity and science intelligence are by no means the same thing, although some degree of scientific comprehension is probably required in order to derive pleasure from seeking out scientific information. However, there is ample evidence to suggest that people who are highly capable of comprehending complex scientific information may be completely uninterested in it and, on the contrary, people who are only vaguely capable of fully understanding complex scientific concepts still get pleasure from seeking out scientific information.

In the study by Kahan and colleagues, subjects were assigned to one of two conditions in which they were confronted with a pair of newspaper headlines, one that was "climate change skeptical" and one that was "climate change non-skeptical." One headline corroborated the notion of human-caused climate change, and the other drew some suspicion about it. Headlines were also characterized as either surprising or unsurprising, emphasizing this as brand new information or reporting it as the status quo. Subjects were instructed to select the headline of most interest to them. The study found that subjects with high levels of science curiosity would consistently engage with headlines that might be opposite their political beliefs if the headline were presented as scientifically novel. Subjects who had low levels of scientific curiosity consistently engaged only with headlines that matched their political views.[59] This means that people were able to overcome their political views if they had high levels of science curiosity and were presented with something scientifically novel.

This study, as well as subsequent research, suggests the importance of piquing people's curiosity in and enjoyment of science, rather than always simply focusing on getting them the right information.[60,61] In fact, getting people the right information without engaging their interest just results in their reaffirming their political and identity-congruent ideas and believing whatever they wanted to believe in the first place. The more we can engage people's interest and curiosity in new scientific concepts, the better chance we have of their being willing to accept new ideas.

In the case of increasing trust in public health officials and healthcare providers, it might be worthwhile to pique people's interest in the science behind the health topics they are looking to make decisions about. This might help steer them away from any political views that might taint a thorough and accurate examination of the facts and help them seek out new information with a more open and perhaps even trusting disposition. Indeed, trust allows for a kind of openness that lends itself well to full scientific inquiry. So a more open inquiry into the nature of a particular health issue and treatments associated with it that is driven by true science curiosity is itself an exercise in increased trust in the system.

Help People See Multiple Sides to Their Identities to Avoid Becoming Mired in Identity Politics

When people focus heavily on their political identities, they are more likely to fall prey to conspiracy theories and misinformation, and it also becomes more difficult for them to consider information that conflicts with what they already believe. This notion makes sense logically because if political identity is your only identity and is the centerpiece of who you are, then information contradicting your preconceived notions will be more threatening than if you have multiple, sometimes internally conflicting identities that allow you to place less weight on any one facet of your identity in particular. When people focus on a variety of components of their identities, rather than fully identifying with a political affiliation, they have an easier time considering conflicting information and changing their minds, in part because they adopt a more flexible mindset.[62] They are, in other words, more open to new data and new information.

People can be encouraged to focus on different parts of their identities by drawing out their interests, concerns, and causes they care about, among other things. Engaging people in a broader conversation about what is generally important to them can help put things in perspective in a way that allows them to be a little less focused on how a certain piece of new information does or does not threaten their politics. This technique is not too different from motivational interviewing, in which you help people focus on their values and goals in order to lead them toward a way of life and a series of decisions that are more congruent with what is most important to them. Deep-seated, unequivocal suspicion of the healthcare system and of healthcare providers is often rooted in conspiratorial thinking styles and ideas that are highly polarized and political. Helping people look outside of their political identities to better understand who they really are can result in an opportunity for the kind of open inquiry that is required for a successful understanding of scientific information.

This chapter has shown that the issue of trust in healthcare and medicine in the general American public is more complex than it seems. While there is certainly a level of distrust that is cause for concern, it is not the case that Americans wholeheartedly distrust the healthcare system. The situation is much more nuanced and can be seen in the general ambivalence of many people about healthcare, their doctors, the health information they consume, and government health agencies. This ambivalence is important to recognize because it forms the basis of many effective interventions that may guide people toward better health decisions that are more in line with their goals and needs. It is therefore not completely accurate to posit that Americans have lost faith in the healthcare system. There are glimmers of hope in the way that Americans feel about doctors, and we have identified ways they can be made to feel more trusting. Again, the function of this exercise is not to teach people to accept everything they hear from doctors and healthcare institutions without question. Distrust in the system is warranted, and a questioning disposition is essential to ensuring that nothing untoward is happening. However, we can teach people to be more discerning of when to be suspicious and when to be more accepting. In the meantime, it is essential to encourage people not to automatically distrust the science behind some of their most important health decisions. After all, it is the duty of public health and medicine to ensure that this often healthy dose of ambivalence does not transform into a wholehearted rejection of the scientific evidence that keeps us safe and healthy.

2

"Othered" Bodies

Medical Mistrust in Black and Latinx Communities

Slavery was no "side-show" in American history—it was the "main event."

—James Oliver Horton, *Slavery and the Making of America*

During a series of focus groups with Black and Latinx communities in 2021, my research team at Critica asked whether participants thought their communities were at greater risk of serious illness and death from COVID-19. Several of the responses from participants in the Black focus group encapsulate the very essence of medical mistrust in marginalized communities that I will expand upon in this chapter. One participant responded:

I feel that my community is more at risk of catching COVID due to the history of us being ignored by health professionals and the government. Additionally, we are most likely in employment opportunities that expose us to conditions that are not ideal. I don't agree that we are experiencing more serious reactions because that implies that we are unhealthy. Unhealthy behaviors are common in America and not assigned to simply one community. If we are having serious reactions, it is most likely due to our concerns being brushed aside when we seek assistance from healthcare workers.

In one breath, this participant discusses both the history of Black Americans and the medical system, as well as the societal and structural features (e.g., employment opportunities that lead to greater exposure) that put Black Americans at greater risk for poor health outcomes, including from COVID-19. This person is especially careful to note that Black people are not inherently less healthy than other communities in the United States ("that implies that we are unhealthy"). This participant appears to have internalized a history of Black bodies being viewed as inherently and medically "different" from White bodies. Another participant said something similar: "I don't feel we are at any higher risk, I feel we don't have access to the best care. Even if we have a good pcp and health system, race and racism can keep us from getting the best care." There is nothing inherent in being Black that produces a greater risk for illness from COVID-19, but rather an ongoing series of social, structural, and cultural factors that lead to significantly worse medical care.

These factors—historical and currently experienced racism in both medical and non-medical settings, social and structural factors related to employment that lead to greater exposure to illnesses and difficulty getting vaccinated, and difficulty accessing quality medical care—are very much at the heart of both the higher risk that Black Americans have consistently faced in the wake of the pandemic and the high rates of medical mistrust in this community. Yet if we take media coverage at face value, we would assume that all Black people are always drawing from one historical event as *the* reason to mistrust the medical establishment: the Tuskegee Syphilis experiment. While it is true that Black Americans look at the example of Tuskegee as a sign not to trust the medical establishment, the layers of mistrust that exist in this community are far more complex than this.

On the one hand, COVID created somewhat of a bridge between White and Black communities, who harbored similar forms of mistrust, especially about the vaccine. On the other hand, the forms of mistrust in Black communities around COVID and the vaccine betray much deeper issues having to do with real experiences of discrimination, dismissal, and poor treatment by medical providers. Furthermore, when considering medical mistrust among minoritized communities, it is important not to conflate communities that have had different historical and social experiences. Forms of medical mistrust in Black and Latinx communities are often conflated in a way that prevents us from seeing the nuances and important differences in the prevailing attitudes in these communities. Medical mistrust in Black communities is often centered around feelings of dismissal and historical concerns about treatments and experimentation without consent, while mistrust in Latinx communities is more closely tied to feelings of uncertainty, related to general concerns about government healthcare services that may have something to do with the immigration experiences common in these communities.

Once again, the important point to note here is that mistrust arises from systemic and structural factors. Instead of "blaming the victim," we must understand the specific societal factors that have raised the level of medical mistrust in Black and Latinx communities—rather than looking to "cultural" factors inherent in these groups to explain it. In some ways, the latter represents the easy way out and allows the rest of American society to shirk responsibility for a very real and very prevalent problem.

Historical Bases of Black Medical Mistrust

The American Medical Association (AMA) Code of Ethics lays out the central role of trust in any doctor-patient therapeutic relationship: "Building relationships of trust with patients is fundamental to ethical practice in medicine.... The relationship between a patient and a physician is based on trust, which gives rise to physicians' ethical responsibility to place patients' welfare above the physician's own self-interest or obligations to others, to use sound medical judgment on patients' behalf, and to advocate for their patients' welfare."[1] Relationships of trust are fundamental to ethical practice in medicine. Without trust, it cannot be said that physicians are putting the interests of their patients first and foremost. It is the responsibility of the physician, not the patient, to ensure that this trust is built.

And yet, beginning with the very first slaves to arrive from Africa in 1619, the relationship between America's medical apparatus and individuals of African descent has been fraught, strained, and at more points than is sometimes fathomable, based on deeply unethical and inhumane medical practices. Throughout American history, Black people have been overly pathologized, abused, subject to unwanted testing and treatment, and at times criminally neglected. At every turn, Black people have been medicalized. During the antebellum period, people talked about "runaway slave syndrome" to "explain" why slaves would flee. Likewise, during the Civil Rights era, some psychiatrists claimed that Black activists were delusional, dangerous, and paranoid as a result of having schizophrenia.[2] Some of the medical technologies we still benefit from today are partially the result of experimentation without consent on Black bodies. For example, J. Marion Sims, widely considered the "father" of modern gynecology, developed vaginal fistula surgery by experimenting on Black female slaves without consent or anesthesia.[3] And of course, there is America's foray into eugenics, with forced sterilization of Black women that lasted until the 1970s.[3]

This shameful, storied history has created a completely understandable and justified veneer of distrust around the medical establishment in Black communities. As Black folklorist John W. Roberts has noted, this history of abuse has created a tendency to tell stories. Sometimes these stories are not entirely accurate, but either way they serve a purpose—to warn about, in his words, "potential dangers or threats to their well-being and survival."[4]

Some scholars have specifically tried to trace medical mistrust in the Black community back to the U.S. Public Health Service (USPHS) Study of Syphilis at Tuskegee. Better known as the "Tuskegee Syphilis Study," this was a clinical study conducted between 1932 and 1972, intended to observe the "natural history" of untreated syphilis infection. Informed consent was not collected and subjects were not offered treatment, even though penicillin was widely available. The study came to an end when an Ad Hoc Advisory Panel convened by the Assistant Secretary for Health and Scientific Affairs recommended it be shut down, and a wide array of media sources published news of this unethical affair for the first time. Six hundred African American men in Macon County, Alabama, were recruited into the study based on a false promise of free healthcare.

Many scholars have sought to understand what the impacts, direct and indirect, have been of this study on Black communities' feelings about and trust in the (mostly White) medical community. This is not an easy phenomenon to quantify, although some studies suggest a rather unsurprising key role of this study in shaping the attitudes of many African American citizens about the trustworthiness of the medical system. Using observational data, Marcella Alsan, a professor of public policy, and economist Marianne Wanamaker have suggested that one-third of the Black-White gap in male life expectancy can be directly traced back to mistrust stemming from Tuskegee.[5] They have suggested that by 1980, the 1972 revelation of Tuskegee had reduced Black life expectancy among Black men over 45 by more than a year.[5] This effect was more common among Black people who were most similar to the subjects of the study (e.g., Black males who lived geographically close by) and among those with community ties to Tuskegee. The authors used data from the General Social Survey to extract information on medical trust, the National Health Interview Survey for data on healthcare utilization, and data from the CDC on morbidity and mortality. The authors note that there were already (and still are) vast differences in health outcomes and utilization rates between White and Black Americans, so they used distance from the epicenter of Tuskegee, demographic similarity to subjects, and migration clusters to determine if health outcomes changed in particular communities with close ties to Tuskegee surrounding the revelation of the study and associated misconduct. Health outcomes, trust, and life expectancy were worse closer to Macon County compared to other surrounding areas. Migrants from Alabama in the aftermath of the revelations of the study still carried worse outcomes and lower trust with them. They did not find the same patterns with younger Black men (versus older Black men), but they were careful to note that this of course does not mean that there are not more current abuses that affect those populations more. These data are of course observational and were not collected as part of the more rigorous experimentation method of a randomized controlled trial, but some of the claims here are compelling nonetheless.

What Alsan and Wanamaker are able to establish here is the presence of something called "group-based medical mistrust." Group-based medical mistrust refers to "a tendency to distrust medical systems and personnel believed to represent the dominant culture in a given society." It is the basis of mistrust especially among marginalized populations who perceive the medical system as belonging to the dominant class in society.[6] The mistrust is therefore immediately cast in terms of power dynamics that have rich cultural and historical underpinnings, as we can witness in the phenomenon of the Tuskegee experiment causing mistrust among Black Americans. Group-based medical mistrust is important in part because it has been shown to have an actual impact on attitudes about seeking care and, often, on help-seeking behaviors. One study, for example, found that high levels of medical mistrust were associated with higher expectations of encountering discrimination in treatment and that these expectations were associated with delays in initiation of treatment (in this study, patients were seeking treatment for addiction).[6]

This group-based medical mistrust and associated expectations of racism and discrimination in medicine have played out in the COVID-19 pandemic, especially surrounding provision of COVID-19 vaccines. In a variety of focus groups conducted by me as well as by other researchers, some participants explicitly mentioned Tuskegee as a reason why they were concerned that the COVID-19 vaccine might have something nefarious in store for Black people in particular (although in our study, it was a minority of participants who mentioned this). Interestingly, one participant in another researcher's focus group was specifically concerned about showing up to the vaccine site and seeing only people of his own race: "Was it just going to be all Black folks in there? And was I going to get back to that thought of, okay they're trying to do something to us, or that we got the contaminated vials.... But when I got in there, seeing the diversity it made me feel better."[7] This comment reveals an interesting reversal of a normal tendency to find comfort in being surrounded by people like us. In this case, there is discomfort in the realization that Black people as a group might be targeted (again) by the medical establishment. Specifically mentioning "contaminated vials," this person is clearly afraid that an act of willful poisoning would occur if he found too many Black people grouped at a vaccination site. This comment betrays a deep-seated medical mistrust that plays out in hesitancy to seek important preventive care against a potentially deadly disease.

Before leaving this section, it is essential to convey the extent to which medical abuses against Black populations were rampant both before and after Tuskegee. Lest readers walk away with the misconception that Tuskegee was the sole (or one of the only) examples of this kind of medical atrocity, let's look at a few other examples (which, even taken together, still do not do justice to the extent of harm caused by a racist medical system against the Black community). In the next section, I will also outline the ways in which other, less obvious factors have caused an entrenched sense of medical mistrust among Black Americans.

There is already some discussion above of forced sterilization, experimentation on Black women to establish vaginal fistula surgery procedures, and the over-pathologization of Black bodies, including the labeling of a new disorder called "runaway slave syndrome." It goes without saying that between 1619 and 1865, Black slaves were consistently used as guinea pigs in numerous inhumane and unethical experiments. What may be more shocking to readers is the fact that some of these forms of unethical experimentation and attitudes toward Black bodies as being disposable continued as part of the medical system almost up until the present day. During the apartheid era in South Africa, South African scientists and leaders worked with assistance from American scientists to develop biowarfare weapons that would selectively target Black people.[8(p378)] From 1981 to 1983, Wouter Basson, a South African cardiologist who was at the time the head of the country's secret chemical and biological warfare program, Project Coast, placed the project under the direction of Daan Goosen, M.D., who was the managing director of Robdeplaat Research Laboratories. About Project Coast, Dr. Goosen told the *Washington Post* that "his division was under orders to perfect agents that would preferentially sabotage blacks' fertility, and to devise a 'silver bullet' biological weapon, designed to kill only black Africans."[8(p378)] American scientists were involved with this research.

Black Americans mostly living in urban areas continued to be experimented on without consent well into the 1990s. In 1956, scientists sought to validate the claim that a particular species of fungus caused lung disease more often in Black people than in White people. The fungus was sprayed across a variety of East Coast cities where more Black people than White people worked at the time. An army report about this incident suggested that the main concern had to do with the potential large-scale "incapacitation" of "employed large numbers of laborers, including many Negroes," whose illness would "seriously affect the operation of the supply system." A Democratic representative from Minnesota, Paul Wellstone, was pivotal in putting a halt to these "experiments," commenting, "No one should ever have been subjected to these tests."[8(p383)] And yet, none of these large-scale biological "experiments" on Black populations in the United States has ever been formally acknowledged by the U.S. government. The equation of Black bodies with elements of the labor "supply system" is eerily reminiscent of the attitude of White Southerners toward Black slaves earlier in American history and, along with this kind of nonconsensual experimentation, suggests continuity from slavery to the present day.

The Baltimore Lead Study conducted by the Johns Hopkins Kennedy Krieger Institute (KKI) is another infamous example of extensive experimentation with limited consent on Black bodies. In this study, KKI targeted Black families in low-income Baltimore neighborhoods to test various degrees of lead abatement strategies. KKI only partially explained the study and potential serious consequences to families, and the result of these forms of partial lead abatement strategies was many cases of serious sequelae from lead exposure among young Black children, many of whom suffered significant cognitive and developmental damage. At the time this study was conducted, there was already a high degree of awareness among scientists that any level of lead is unsafe for young children, so deliberately exposing children to lead that was only partially abated is a serious ethical breach. Not fully explaining the potential consequences, which included neurological damage, to parents was another serious ethical breach. The full public understanding of the study and subsequent legal action did not occur until the early 2000s, in very recent memory.

Medical Mistrust and Ambivalence Among Black Americans

There is no question that the history of Black Americans in the United States is indescribably sullied by numerous examples of scientific and medical abuses, the most famous of which is probably the Tuskegee Syphilis Study. These examples of egregious scientific misconduct have undoubtedly contributed to the relatively low levels of medical and scientific trust in Black communities that persist to this day. However, I would be remiss if I assigned Black medical mistrust to the sole cause of medical abuses that exist in the past. For one thing, this kind of argument suggests that the causes of Black medical mistrust are linked to occurrences that happened to "other" people, rather than recognizing that certain types of abuses, though perhaps subtler, persist. In addition, when we assign all the blame to events of the past, we implicitly place the burden of emerging from this form of mistrust on the affected party. In other words, by suggesting that Black medical mistrust persists because of events in the past, we are implying that in order to get out of this pattern of suspicion, Black communities must ultimately learn to put the past behind them. This, in a way, absolves White Americans and does not fully allow them to recognize the damage they continue to do.

On the other hand, if we recognize that the persistence of medical mistrust in these communities is based largely on contemporary experiences of discrimination, racism, and, importantly, poor access to often lower-quality care, then the story becomes much more complex. No longer can we assert that the path to a more positive sentiment about healthcare lies in the hands of Black Americans, who must learn to adjust their expectations and recover from the trauma of decades-old abuses. The "blame" in this instance shifts more squarely onto the healthcare system itself, calling for systemic, often radical reforms that could hopefully result in more equitable outcomes.

In her seminal work on race and medicine, *Medical Apartheid*, Harriet Washington commented on the noted disparity in the 1990s between Black and White uptake of the first medication for HIV/AIDS, zidovudine (originally known as AZT):

> Misguided research has caused HIV therapy to be withheld from blacks even as it has heavily ladled guilt for the spread of AIDS upon their shoulders. For example, in the early 1990s, a Johns Hopkins study revealed that HIV-positive whites, but not blacks, were doubling their survival

time by taking AZT. Conventional wisdom has long laid this disparity at the feet of African Americans by insisting that blacks resisted taking AZT . . . because of fear and distrust engendered by the U.S. PHS syphilis study at Tuskegee.[8(p340)]

Washington's observation here is spot on. Focusing on Tuskegee as a reason for low uptake of HIV therapy places a kind of blame on Black people, ultimately for continuing to spread the disease.

Washington goes on to observe that:

With a singular myopia, scientific and social science researchers have ignored the appalling wealth of other pharmaceutical and infectious-disease experimentation with blacks to seize instead upon a single PHS study with very imperfect parallels to the HIV crisis. Celebrated surveys did not ask open-ended questions to determine the roots of black aversion to AZT; instead, they asked specifically whether the Tuskegee Syphilis Study was "the" factor. Popular coverage widely conveyed the assumption that the emotional overreaction of blacks to this single investigation abuse was at fault. But this monomaniac focus upon the Tuskegee Syphilis Study as the catalyst for AZT aversion ignores some pertinent research history.[8]

This obsession with Tuskegee, as she calls it, a "single PHS study with very imperfect parallels" to other situations such as the HIV crisis, creates a "myopia" that disincentivizes any examination of other factors that might contribute to Black medical mistrust. Feeling as though they have "found the answer," many social scientists still stop at Tuskegee as *the* explanation for Black communities' hesitancy surrounding modern medical care. This is misguided, not least because it shirks responsibility for continuing discrimination and episodes of abuse, but also because it mischaracterizes the true nature of Black medical mistrust in the modern era. There is reason to believe that while Tuskegee is *a* factor in this mistrust, it is not *the only* factor upon which we should lay our narrative of medical mistrust in this population. As Washington hints, one key to getting closer to a more accurate understanding of the drivers of medical hesitancy in Black communities is asking "open-ended questions," allowing Black participants to fully voice their opinions on this topic, rather than giving them closed surveys that more often than not explicitly evoke thoughts about Tuskegee. While Washington focuses on other pertinent research abuses similar to Tuskegee that drive medical mistrust, I will spend the next portion of this chapter focusing more closely on structural and sociopolitical factors that have created a pervasive feeling of firm ambivalence in Black communities about the extent to which the medical system has its members' best interests at heart.

Systemic distrust extends beyond the healthcare system, and there is evidence that distrust of other institutions can affect people's attitudes about health and medicine. Black communities "do not trust systems that are connected to white supremacy."[9] While some might feel that connecting the modern healthcare system to White supremacy is a bridge too far, there are two reasons why this connection is valid. One is the horrific history, narrated so well by Harriet Washington, of the medical system's perpetration of abuses on Black bodies, many examples of which still occurred in very recent memory. Second, our healthcare system is still highly segregated, as demonstrated not only by the often separate services available for White and Black communities, but also by a pervasive view in the medical community that health among Black people and White people is fundamentally different.

Vanessa Northington Gamble, a giant in the field of medical mistrust, particularly in the Black community, has drawn an important distinction between "trust" and "trustworthiness." As she notes, by focusing so much on the trust or mistrust of Black people in the medical system, we put the onus on them to change their views and be more "trusting." But it is the responsibility of the healthcare system to engender "trustworthiness." In other words, the institutions that comprise the healthcare system have to take action to make themselves worthy of the trust of a community that not only has been historically abused by them, but that still experiences high degrees of racism and discrimination in everyday interactions with healthcare providers and the system surrounding them.[10-14]

The various ways in which the healthcare system treats Black people as though they are "different" are some of the most problematic components of the relationship between Black communities and healthcare in this country. The way we all, including the medical community, talk about health disparities can sometimes exacerbate a sense of division that engenders more mistrust. As Gamble points out, "There is a long history of Black bodies being seen as different within the medical sphere, that Black bodies are inferior, that Black people are susceptible to particular disease because of their bodies."[15] This notion is still alive and well when we talk about Black people being more susceptible to serious COVID-19 disease due to a higher frequency of underlying conditions, such as hypertension and diabetes. While it is true that the prevalence of these illnesses is higher in the Black community, there is hardly ever discussion of why this is and how much this might have to do with our social and medical systems that create the conditions for Black people to be more susceptible to these diseases in the first place. These conditions include factors such as food deserts, living in areas with high levels of pollution and other environmental harms, and lack of access to preventive healthcare, among other factors. And then, of course, as a result of having higher rates of chronic diseases, they are more prone to getting sicker with a novel antigen such as COVID-19.

This view of Black and White bodies as fundamentally different is not new. It was always a common sentiment to view Black bodies as inferior to White bodies. This was very often the explanation for any kind of elevated incidence of disease among Black people compared to White people. At the end of the Civil War, for example, there was a high incidence of tuberculosis in the Black community. The medical community reasoned that this had to do with their "inferior" constitution.[15] When we only talk about the disparities and make no mention of the surrounding social and environmental conditions, we tap into this legacy of Black body "inferiority."

So the medical system's continuing tendency to draw differences between White and Black bodies, as well as its general hesitancy to fully own its current role in racism and discrimination in healthcare, engenders greater degrees of mistrust in the Black community. Indeed, we have plenty of examples of Black people seeking medical care who are less interested in historical incidences such as Tuskegee and more concerned about everyday issues such as access challenges, perceived racism and discrimination, and general concerns about being treated differently or being put in a racially motivated category. Karen Lincoln, a professor of social work at University of Southern California (USC) said that when she asks Black seniors in Los Angeles about the COVID vaccine, Tuskegee rarely comes up. This is even among elderly members of the Black community, who might arguably have more recent ties to the infamous "experiment."[16] To her, it is mainly academics and public officials who are preoccupied with Tuskegee, not members of the community.

Epidemiologist Ralph Katz was also skeptical of the firm line that both scholars and especially public media have been drawing between Tuskegee and the modern-day hesitancy to seek medical care and participate in biomedical research studies among Black Americans. He decided to put the notion to the test, specifically looking at refusal to participate in research because of the legacy of Tuskegee. He found that while Black participants in his study were twice as likely as White participants to admit being "wary" of participating in biomedical research studies, they were equally likely to report being willing to participate and there was no association between knowledge of or feelings about Tuskegee and the level of willingness.[16] To be clear, he found a lot of hesitancy among Black participants, but not necessarily outright refusal. It is also more likely that this hesitancy had to do with factors outside of Tuskegee.

Maxine Toler, a 72-year-old president of her city's senior advocacy council, told the *LA Times* that when she asks other Black seniors in her neighborhood about Tuskegee, they often have only a vague notion of what actually happened. They are, she says, "fuzzy" on the details.[16] When asked about COVID and any potential connection to Tuskegee that the situation might be calling up in people's minds, Ms. Toler responded that she thought: "It's almost the opposite of Tuskegee. Because they were being denied treatment. And this is like, we're pushing people forward: Go and get this vaccine. We want everybody to be protected from COVID."[16] While perhaps not exactly the "opposite" of COVID, there is a firm suggestion here that perhaps Black communities are not using the collective memory of Tuskegee to make decisions about health and trust in healthcare in the way many researchers think they are. Perhaps Tuskegee is part of a historical legacy that helps make sense of today's continued inequities, but it is not likely to be the primary driver of medical mistrust among most Black people.

The true story of modern-day Black medical mistrust is in fact more complex than the horrific memory of Tuskegee's abuse of research subjects. We may even be able to detect some of the ambivalence about health and healthcare professionals, a kind of uncertain trust, of the sort I discussed in Chapter 1. Aside from shedding light on some Black people's memories of Tuskegee, Toler also shared an important insight about the various ways that the COVID-19 pandemic and the situation with the vaccine in the early days right after it was approved might have contributed to medical mistrust in the Black community. At the same time that Black people were being especially encouraged to get the vaccine due to the "high-risk" nature of many in Black communities, they were finding it especially difficult to access. Access issues that were seen in non-Black communities were exacerbated in Black communities, not least because the primary way to get an appointment was to sit on a computer all day and continuously refresh the page, a luxury many members of the Black community do not have. As Toler mentions, trying to get the vaccine and yet not having access to it actually sowed mistrust in the healthcare system.[16] It may or may not be true that vaccine hesitancy has been higher in Black communities, but there is a strong clue in Toler's comments: access issues plant the seed for medical mistrust, and we know that access is an enduring problem in Black communities. That poor access leads to medical mistrust is a major argument of this book, and there is no reason to believe minority populations are any different.

In fact, perceived discrimination in healthcare situations may dictate a lot of medical mistrust, but the discrimination does not necessarily have to be about race or ethnicity, even among minority populations. One recent study found that having a higher level of perceived discrimination due to income or type of insurance increased the odds of research participants responding "not at all or not enough trust" in healthcare providers and the healthcare system by 98%.[17] This study found a closer association between high levels of perceived discrimination around income and lack of insurance and medical mistrust than between perceived discrimination around race or ethnicity and medical trust—and this is by no means the first study to find this.[17-20] In general, there are findings in the literature that strongly suggest that Medicaid recipients have some of the highest levels of suspicion of the healthcare system of anyone.[21,22]

The authors note, importantly, that, controlling for everything else (including race and ethnicity), the greatest predictor of medical mistrust was not having a primary care provider. Individuals without primary care providers, regardless of perceived discrimination of various kinds, insurance status, income level, race, ethnicity, gender, and numerous other factors, had 7 times the rate of reporting high levels of mistrust in providers and the healthcare system compared to individuals who did have a primary care provider. The authors go on to note that COVID-19 may have made hard-to-reach populations even harder to reach. Many people who did not have an existing relationship with a primary care provider, who may have, according to them, higher levels of medical mistrust, were unable to reach anyone via telehealth, as many providers were seeing only existing patients this way. This increased difficulty in gaining access to healthcare can exacerbate trust even under normal circumstances. Add to that the fact that we were (and still are) in the midst of an unprecedented health crisis full of confusing new information and directives that began under the leadership of a very right-wing, often racist administration, and it is not hard to see why people's mistrust increased.

This is most certainly not to say that perceived racial or ethnic discrimination is *not* a factor in medical mistrust. It is just not the *only* factor, even for people from minority racial and ethnic groups. A more recent study from 2022 found that there is a strong association with perceived lack of general support from a healthcare provider and anticipation of upcoming racial discrimination. That is, people who felt unsupported or perhaps even unseen by their healthcare providers assumed that racial discrimination would almost naturally be a part of future interactions.[6] In the same study, there was also a moderate correlation between a perception of health disparities and anticipation of racial discrimination during treatment, which often led to delayed care-seeking. In the study, which looked at people in treatment for drug addiction, there was a strong association between a reported history of racial discrimination in healthcare and anticipation of future racial discrimination during treatment and moderate correlation with delayed care-seeking. History of racial discrimination and the suspicion subscale were ultimately the two factors most strongly correlated with anticipation of racial discrimination during addiction treatment. History of racial discrimination in healthcare and an inclination toward generally suspicious attitudes as correlates of medical mistrust and anticipation of future discrimination are perhaps not the most surprising findings. But the notion that perception of future discrimination might be at least in part dictated by a sense of lack of support from healthcare providers and perceptions of health disparities is extremely important. It suggests that these expectations are malleable based on the quality of interactions with healthcare providers, even if there is a history of discrimination. In other words, positive trust-building interactions with clinicians can lessen suspicious attitudes.

The mistreatment that many Black patients face is often perpetuated by healthcare providers' discriminatory attitudes about the extent to which Black patients are "compliant" or "noncompliant." The implicit bias against this group of patients has been studied in part by looking at medical records. It is much more common to see words such as "belligerent," "unwilling," "noncompliant," "refused," and "difficult patient" in doctors' notes about non-Hispanic Black patients than about non-Hispanic White patients.[23] In one study, Black patients had 2.54 the odds of having a negative descriptor in their electronic health record (EHR) compared with White patients.[24] The combination of general lack of reliable access to quality healthcare and an atmosphere in which providers assume that Black patients are difficult and noncompliant creates a perfect scenario for mistrust to flourish.

Some subset of Black patients will always internalize providers' assumptions about noncompliance and struggle with important health behaviors such as medication adherence partially as a result. It is difficult to know exactly what goes into the provider's calculation who assumes that Black patients are more likely to be noncompliant than White patients, in part because many providers may be unaware that they hold this assumption in the first place. It is likely a combination of flat-out bias, perhaps holding Black patients to a different standard than White patients (e.g., deciding that they are "difficult" if they ask more than a few questions, when this behavior would be considered normal in a White patient), and an internalized racially biased legacy in medicine in which Black patients were expected to be silent and comply without protest to a wide array of experiments and procedures. This third factor is likely to be buried in the minds of most providers, who would not believe that they may have internalized certain implicit messages from their medical training that have created unrealistic expectations of Black patients in particular.

Sometimes mistrust leads the way to more extreme thinking as well. Conspiracy theories are no more common in the Black community than in other racial groups in the United States per se, but there are a lot of medical conspiracy theories surrounding HIV/AIDS to which a sizable proportion of people subscribe. In one study, 27% of African Americans believed that "HIV/AIDS is a man-made virus that the federal government made to kill and wipe out Black people."[25] Twenty-seven percent is a minority, albeit a substantial one, but the statement is also quite extreme, so the fact that this many people agreed with it is not insignificant. Similarly, over 20% of African American women believed that AIDS was made in a government laboratory.

Interestingly in this study, high levels of belief in HIV conspiracy theories were not necessarily associated with high levels of medical mistrust. It is possible that these beliefs were more bound to distrust of government than distrust of healthcare providers and the healthcare system, and that these levels of trust are kept separate in people's minds. Nonetheless, we do know that conspiracy beliefs relate to wider social and intergroup conflicts and are often used in instances that involve a perceived lack of control and psychological empowerment or to attribute blame to an unjust social system. Feelings of helplessness are also highly correlated with conspiracy beliefs in specific communities.[25] Given the not insignificant level of belief in HIV-related conspiracy beliefs, it is essential to remember that Black communities continue to deal with a major health crisis that is associated with distrust of the government, feelings of disempowerment and helplessness, and even some extreme conspiracy beliefs. While the average Black community member does not harbor the same level of conspiracy beliefs about COVID-19, some of the feelings about trusting (or not trusting) the government and feelings of disempowerment might be similar across COVID-19 and HIV/AIDS-related conspiracy theories.

Unfortunately, healthcare is not the only institutional locus in which Black people experience racism and discrimination. An array of studies has tried to better understand the relationships among medical mistrust and conspiracy theories, structural discrimination, and perceptions and experiences of everyday racism and discrimination. One study from 2019 found that reported experiences of everyday racism and discrimination, even if they did not occur in the healthcare arena, were associated with delays in certain health-seeking behaviors, including preventive screenings and routine checkups.[26] Both everyday discrimination and, perhaps not surprisingly, healthcare discrimination more specifically were associated with greater degrees of medical mistrust and endorsing medical conspiracy theories. However, in another, more recent study, experiences of structural discrimination did not increase medical mistrust and medical conspiracy theorizing.[27] It is difficult to know what would drive such a difference here, and it's important to note that measuring the relationship between sweeping institutional discrimination and distrust of the healthcare system is not easy. It's still possible, and perhaps likely, that structural discrimination is also a driver of medical mistrust and conspiracy theories. It's also possible that interpersonal mistrust carries over from one arena to another more easily than institutional mistrust, such that experiences of everyday racism and discrimination on an interpersonal level might lead to avoiding interpersonal interactions in a healthcare setting as well.

Just how often do Black patients report encountering racism and discrimination in healthcare environments? In a recent Kaiser Family Foundation poll, 7 in 10 Black Americans reported believing that race-based discrimination in healthcare happens at least somewhat often, and 1 in 5 say they've experienced it themselves in the past year.[28] When asked about negative experiences, the number is more comparable to the rest of the American population, at around 55%.[29] In the classic tome *An American Health Dilemma*, Linda Clayton and Michael Byrd trace this legacy quite elegantly from the antebellum period all the way to the new millennium. They argue that there is an enduring professional assumption that Black health is somehow inherently "poor health":

> The professional assumption of poor health as "normal" for Blacks remained ingrained in the minds of White American physicians—who went so far as to create a lexicon of "Negro diseases" and alternate physiological mechanisms based on race—well into the twentieth century. All these factors aggravated and perpetuated the pattern of inferior, inconstant, or unavailable health care for people of African descent in the United States.[30]

In the late 19th and 20th centuries, numerous treatises were written that sought to uncover and explain this "difference" between White and Black bodies. In the process,

> [t]he decline in already poor Black health was blamed on African Americans' self-destructive behavioral traits, immoral behavior, weak constitutions, inherent susceptibility to disease, distaste for labor, criminality, fondness for alcohol, disregard for personal hygiene, ignorance of laws of nutrition, and proclivity for sexual vices and immorality. This climate of biological and scientific racism, along with the physical and legal atrocities being committed against Black citizens served as the social setting and atmosphere in which the late nineteenth-century and early twentieth-century American hospital and medical education reform movements occurred.[30]

This legacy continued despite a short-term improvement in minority health status between 1965 and 1975. As Byrd and Clayton argue, this was a "Civil Rights era in healthcare." During this period, Black people made real gains in "virtually all indicators measuring health status, health outcomes, health services, and representation and participation in the health professions." A lot of this was already over by 1975, when, as Byrd and Clayton argue, White enthusiasm for "righting long-term wrongs and inadequacies" petered out. Once Reagan was president, socially regressive policies became the norm in many arenas, including healthcare and health disparities. His administration cut back on entitlement programs such as Medicaid and Medicare that were important for access for Black and other minority populations.

Not long after, the health maintenance organization (HMO) managed-care movement took over in the 1980s and 1990s. Byrd and Clayton argue that this movement was particularly detrimental to Black communities. Part of the movement here was to enroll Medicaid patients into HMOs, which have a heavy focus on cutting costs, restriction of services, and service denial. It has been argued that the HMO managed-care legacy continues into the present day, with Black patients regularly facing severe restrictions on their utilization of healthcare services. It is not hard to understand why Clayton and Byrd draw a straight line between certain political realities and legacies in this country and the health status and attitudes about healthcare among Black patients. Indeed, there is much to be said for an argument that puts American obsession with marketplace economics and "rugged individualism" at the center of the problem of Black access to care and subsequent medical mistrust. This line of argument suggests we must take a wide lens to truly understand the nature of medical mistrust in Black and other minority populations. Part of the story is the horrific treatment of Black communities throughout history in the name of medicine and science. Part of the story is the legacy of a healthcare system and set of practices that always placed a rift between White and Black bodies. And equally part of the story is a political system that favors the well-being of the individual over that of larger communities and populations and relies on marketplace economics to create a "fair" system of access and treatment. We should resist the urge to tell a completely separate story about Black medical mistrust, because while there is a specific history of abuse and mistreatment of this population, it is also the case that Black medical mistrust is intimately connected to a variety of American political and socioeconomic factors that have created access issues that are at the center of many patients'—Black and not Black—hesitancy about the healthcare system.

COVID-19 and Medical Mistrust in Black Communities

So much of the recent scholarly literature on and media coverage of Black medical mistrust focuses on COVID-19. There have been many attempts to tie vaccine hesitancy in Black communities back to atrocities such as Tuskegee and to understand current medical mistrust in light of past abuses. As I have argued throughout this chapter, while abuses like Tuskegee are certainly part of the story, they do not give a full picture of the rich, complex set of reasons behind modern-day medical mistrust in Black communities. This is not different in the case of COVID-19. Hesitancy around the COVID vaccines in Black communities draws from Tuskegee and other historical examples to a certain extent, but there are also a wide range of other reasons for mistrust and hesitancy, some of which are very similar to what we see in White communities. In some ways, the shared trauma and uncertainty around COVID-19 have created somewhat of a bridge between the types of hesitancy and mistrust we see in White communities and what we see in Black communities. In studies done by me as well as others, it's very apparent that Black patients are hesitant for many of the same reasons that White patients are, not least because of the novelty of the illness and the vaccines and concern over potential long-term side effects that have not been discovered yet.

As one Black 45-year-old mathematics teacher in Pennsylvania put it, the decision to get vaccinated is simply an emotional one in many ways: "Trust is based on emotions, and I just don't trust right now. . . . I'm educated. I have a graduate degree. I read a lot. I'm informed. I'm not a person who clings to conspiracy theories, but I simply do not trust the government at this point."[31(np)] Trust in the government and in the health and medical systems that created and distribute the vaccines is obviously a complex phenomenon based on a wide array of factors, and the COVID-19 crisis has only brought this into even sharper relief. It has highlighted the places where Black Americans' mistrust is similar to White Americans' mistrust and the equally important ways in which it is quite different.

So far, media coverage has focused extensively on vaccine hesitancy specifically in the Black community. There is some discussion of access issues, but this is less prominent in the story the media are telling.[32] Many surveys suggest that Black Americans are not the most vaccine-hesitant of the general population, at least when it comes to the COVID vaccine, and even when they are more hesitant in certain surveys, it may not be by that much.[32] It is possible that many media sources are telling an exaggerated story about the extent of hesitancy in this population. This is a problem because social norming is a very real phenomenon when it comes to decisions about vaccines; that is, people will make decisions about whether to get a vaccine based on their perception of how many other people in their community are getting them. So a false pretense of excessive vaccine hesitancy in Black communities might dissuade some Black people from getting the vaccine.

In focus groups conducted with Black Americans to better understand attitudes toward the COVID vaccine, some participants placed strong emphasis on the ability to make choices as part of the vaccine experience. One participant appreciated having a choice of which vaccine to get: "There was a list of the different vaccines, and I checked the one I wanted. . . . I had a choice definitely for what I signed up for."[7] Another participant noted having some freedom of choice of which lane to pick at a vaccination site: "They didn't just say okay you go to this person. When the lanes opened up . . . they were like, just pick a lane . . . it just made me feel relieved that I had a choice of which lane I could go to. It wasn't just like go to the back of the room."[7] This element of choice is important to everyone, but it is not surprising that it might be particularly important to Black communities given the history discussed in this chapter. While this may not have been a conscious thought for these focus group participants, Black people may feel they have limited choices in the current healthcare environment, which can engender a feeling of mistrust. Even small gestures, such as letting people choose which spot they go to at a vaccination site, can help foster a sense of empowerment and self-efficacy that contributes to trust. While this is obviously not in any way an adequate solution to some of the deep-seated reasons for Black medical mistrust, it is a small step that health centers and other healthcare-providing institutions can take to make matters better in the meantime.

When it comes to reasons for vaccine hesitancy in Black versus White communities, the results are often somewhat mixed. One of the biggest reasons for both Black and White communities to be hesitant about the vaccine is safety concerns. In one study, 39% of Black participants cited safety concerns as the chief reason for being uncertain about the vaccine versus a very similar 40% among White participants. However, a close second for Black participants was mistrust of the government and the healthcare system (32%), a figure that was lower among White participants (23%).[33] White participants were much more likely than Black participants to say they did not think they wanted or needed a vaccine and they were not likely to get sick from COVID (39% versus 21%).[28] In a sense, COVID created a bridge between White and Black medical mistrust, in which many of the reasons for vaccine hesitancy were similar or the same. However, we should be careful not to overlook the underlying feelings of uncertainty about the trustworthiness of both the government and the healthcare system that may have been stronger motivators in decisions about the vaccine for Black than for White communities. We should also note that mistrust of the government and mistrust of the healthcare system, while sharing some features, are not exactly the same phenomenon and that the historical, social, cultural, and political underpinnings of governmental mistrust and medical mistrust are somewhat distinct. These differences will be discussed at greater length in Chapter 5.

Medical Mistrust in Latinx Communities: The Role of Fear and Uncertainty

Historically, medical mistrust in Latinx communities is an understudied topic, especially compared to the same phenomenon in Black communities. When the two are studied together, a lot often gets elided, creating a picture of similarly disadvantaged and abused populations that have similar reasons for mistrust. Yet when we look at data from surveys on mistrust, the two populations are not always aligned. Hesitancy about the COVID-19 vaccine is a good example of this. Latinx participants were often in the middle, showing more distrust and hesitancy than White participants but less than Black participants. For example, a systematic review of studies on COVID-19 vaccine hesitancy found pooled prevalence of vaccine hesitancy of 26.3% among White Americans, 30.2% among Latinx Americans, and 41.6% among Black Americans.[34]

In more in-depth studies of Latinx vaccine hesitancy, researchers have found some of the following elements to be key in concerns about the vaccine: potential long-term side effects (79%); that the vaccine would be ineffective (68%); danger given existing health conditions (62%); not trusting the Trump administration (61%); and expense (60%). Some of these concerns are similar to concerns of the White population, especially around side effects and efficacy. But the high distrust of the Trump administration specifically calls to mind something else that has affected Latinx communities in their trust of the healthcare system and the government: immigration status. While many minority groups in the United States had reason to thoroughly distrust the Trump administration, evidence from other studies that Latinx communities were concerned that the government-sponsored administration of the vaccine might somehow result in negative consequences for undocumented people suggests that this distrust of the administration ranks so high on the list because this is a primary concern.[35] Indeed, some Latinx communities have expressed explicit concern about getting their children tested for COVID, for fear that the government would take away any children who tested positive.[36] In a recent focus group study in which Latinx participants were asked about

their attitudes and intentions about the COVID-19 vaccine, one participant said:

> When hearing about the plan to prioritize minorities, I'm afraid. We never
> know if Trump is involved. I think we need much more information and
> understand why we should be first [to receive the vaccine]. We are very re-
> sistant people. The OHA [Oregon Health Authority] are trying to help us
> be the priority. Their intentions are good. But we have doubts about this
> President; we think about how Trump is.[37]

Others agreed that "prioritizing minority people will cause mistrust."[37]
The concerns about the Trump administration and fears about having children taken away from them suggest that Latinx communities are responding
to the COVID-19 vaccine through the lens of recent trauma under the
Trump administration. They have active concerns about how receiving a
vaccine distributed by the government and getting tests whose results will be
reported to governmental institutions in many cases will affect their immigration status and that of their children. This ongoing fear and uncertainty
about immigration is in many ways the backdrop to their medical mistrust
and hesitancy. While the resulting mistrust is similar to that of the Black
community, the historical, political, and social legacy is not exactly the same
and needs to be examined on its own terms.

There is a lack of research on medical mistrust in this population, and the
scales normally used for these purposes have not been specifically validated
in Latinx people.[17,38] In the studies that do exist, Latinx communities report
a significant amount of discrimination in healthcare settings, although they
attribute most of it to language barriers as opposed to race or ethnicity, income, and insurance status, which are the major perceived drivers of discrimination in the Black population.[17] Latinx communities have good
reason to be skeptical, in light of a history of abuses in the United States in
the name of medical science. In the 1950s, for example, Puerto Rican women
from low-income communities were given experimental birth control pills
without being told they were in a trial.[39] Beginning in 1946, the U.S. government intentionally infected 5,000 people in Guatemala with the bacteria
that causes syphilis in order to study the disease.[40] There is no shortage of
examples like this.

Still, as we have seen from the example of Black communities, it is important not to assume the underlying causes of medical mistrust in any

population and to investigate it in earnest. In several studies conducted over the course of the pandemic, Latinx communities seem slightly less hesitant about the vaccine than Black communities. In a 2021 study, about half as many Black as White people said they would get the vaccine, but the difference between Latinx and White people was not significant.[41] White participants and Latinx participants were equally as likely to say they would recommend the vaccine to family and friends (around 50% each), but Black participants were significantly less likely (32.3%).[41] On the other hand, both Black and Latinx participants were significantly less likely than White participants to say they would get the vaccine right away (20.1% for Black participants, 28.2% for Latinx participants, 38.5% for White participants).[41]

A 2020 study conducted by Kaiser Family Foundation had similar findings—Latinx participants were often either in between Black and White participants or closer to White participants in many of their attitudes toward the vaccine and medicine more generally. At that point, half of Black participants said they would get the vaccine versus 60% of Latinx participants and 65% of White participants.[28] Only 17% of Black participants said they would "definitely" get the vaccine versus 37% of both White and Latinx respondents. Black adults were 19 percentage points less likely than White adults to trust doctors, 14 percentage points less likely to trust hospitals, and 11 percentage points less likely to trust the healthcare system. Latinx adults were always between Black and White adults on this one.[28]

These statistics may not be the absolute best barometer of current attitudes toward the vaccine for various reasons, including sampling difficulties and the fact that at least one of them was conducted before the vaccines were widely available. Nonetheless, they do suggest that we should be careful about assuming Latinx communities have the same attitudes as Black communities simply because there are similar histories of medical abuse. The legacies of these populations in this country and their cultural heritage are distinct, and we should not lose sight of that as we attempt to understand their feelings of trust (or lack of them) toward medicine and the healthcare system.

The Complexity of Trust in Black and Latinx Communities

What I hope to have argued throughout this chapter is that the picture of medical mistrust in Black and Latinx populations is much more complicated than has previously been posited. Trust is very much on a continuum, and the height of ambivalence is in the middle, where mistrust often sits. People in a state of mistrust are mainly *unsure* about whether or not they can trust someone or something. This turns out to be a highly accurate way to describe current Black and Latinx attitudes toward the healthcare system.

In addition, the historical legacy of horrific events such as the Tuskegee and Guatemala syphilis studies must be placed in appropriate context. These events influence overall feelings about the healthcare system in Black and Latinx populations, but they do not dictate levels of trust in these communities. Moreover, they increase and decrease along with certain demographic factors, such as age and proximity to the location of the historical abuse. Modern factors such as access, insurance status, socioeconomic status, and real and perceived episodes of both structural discrimination and everyday racism play a major role in contemporary levels of trust among Black and Latinx communities. This suggests the need for a more sophisticated response than simply raising physicians' awareness of the historical legacy of medical abuse against these populations.

It is equally important to understand mistrust in populations as separate phenomena. It is common to see Black and Latinx populations conflated in discussions of mistrust stemming from past medical abuse. While it is true that medical abuses were perpetrated against these populations, they also have very distinct cultural, historical, and social legacies in this country, as well as differing social structures and value systems that make amalgamating them for the purposes of defining medical mistrust in "minority" populations questionable. Their attitudes and fears need to be separated out and studied in their own right.

A variety of "solutions" to the problem of medical mistrust in Black, Latinx, and other minority populations have already been proposed. I do think that greater attention to medical mistrust and potential signs of it in medical education could be useful, especially if physicians-to-be gain a better understanding of the types of discrimination that minority populations are most prone to or expecting, including not only everyday racism, but also discrimination based on socioeconomic and insurance status. In this case, it is possible that physicians are simply unaware of the extent to which a sense of different treatment based on these circumstances might lead to a feeling of mistrust. It has also often been proposed that an emphasis on implicit bias in both medical training and continuing medical education would be an important element here. Some states have already passed mandatory implicit bias training in medical education.[42] While it probably would not hurt, I do not believe that implicit bias training is necessarily the answer here, and I would hate to see medical education committees thinking they have "solved" the problem based on implementing these trainings alone. While better awareness of how we are communicating our biases, even when unbeknownst to us, will likely help matters, there is no strong evidence that these kinds of trainings actually result in lower levels of mistrust in the populations in which we are interested.[43] Until we see that kind of data, it is difficult to advance this as such a promising answer to the problem of medical mistrust.

In fact, there is generally a dearth of good evidence in terms of what works to increase medical trust in Black and Latinx communities. Many have suggested the importance of race concordance, that is, seeing a doctor or nurse who is your same race or ethnicity. A 2018 study suggested that it isn't just the fact of seeing a Black doctor that might improve the treatment experience, but something about the value of the communication in a race-concordant dyad that might be better than that in a race-discordant dyad.[44] In this study, Black participants were given pictures of their doctors, some White and some Black, and then asked whether they would agree to certain preventive care measures (such as immunizations, screenings, etc.). In this group, those assigned to a photo of a Black doctor were no more likely than those assigned to a photo of a White doctor to indicate intention to receive preventive care. Once participants actually saw and spoke to doctors, however, those assigned to a Black doctor were 18 percentage points more likely to indicate intention to receive preventive care compared to those assigned to a White doctor. The authors conclude that there is something about the communication that takes place between the race-concordant dyad that likely creates a sense of trust and greater engagement in care, but that just the fact of seeing a Black doctor on its own is not the driver behind this finding. This finding was bolstered by surveys of 1,490 people, in which the authors found that when asked about who was the most qualified, both Black and White respondents picked race-concordant doctors about 50% of the time, but when asked who had the best communication, this jumped to 65% for Black respondents and 70% for White respondents.[44] This study would suggest that there might be reason to believe that increasing diversity in the medical profession might help with medical trust.

In terms of right now and our major concern about getting more people vaccinated against COVID-19, one measure we must absolutely take is to stop singling out Black and Latinx communities as particularly hesitant to the vaccine. It is true that there is a lot of mistrust and suspicion in these communities, attitudes that are warranted in many cases. There are also greater access issues, which perpetuate mistrust. And in the case of Latinx communities, there are very real and very disturbing underlying fears about immigration and real trauma from what the Trump administration did to Latinx immigrants and their children and families. All of this is reflected in the published literature thus far about vaccine hesitancy in these communities and in the research conducted by my team at Critica. What is harder to get a sense of is what harping on these communities as hesitant does to attitudes toward them among other communities, as well as damage to the goal of getting more people vaccinated.

On the first point, harping on hesitancy in Black and Latinx communities creates a perception that these populations are somehow to blame for lower vaccine coverage and poorer health outcomes. Nothing could be further from the truth. This "hesitancy," if we should even call it that, arises from a complex patchwork of historical legacy and contemporary social, cultural, and political realities that conspire to create a sense of completely understandable and justified mistrust in these populations. On top of that, there are very real access issues that should not be overlooked, not least because they contribute to mistrust and hesitancy. It is not even clear that rates of vaccination are that much lower in these communities, or that attitudes are overall that much more hesitant (there is a lot of hesitancy among White communities now), and even if they were, we cannot judge off the cuff but must understand the deeply complex and often very disturbing history of Black and Latinx medical care and research in this country to get a better sense of why these attitudes might be arising. It would be difficult, after understanding that history and current access issues, to frame this as certain populations just being in some way "ignorant" or less "willing" to believe in and trust the vaccine. That would be akin to blaming health disparities, which carry with them a centuries-old legacy of historical abuse and disempowerment, on the populations that suffer them.

On the second point, we have to be more sensitive to the reality of "social norming" as a powerful driver of behavior. Studies have repeatedly shown that the behavior of people in close proximity with whom we identify is a powerful motivator of our own behavior. This concept of "peer benchmarking" has helped lower energy use[45–47] and has stopped physicians from doing unnecessary procedures.[48–51] It is also the case that even the perception of the behavior of those we deem similar to us, who are part of our social group, can influence our behavior as well. This has been demonstrated especially convincingly in studies of teen substance use behavior.[52,53] It is not terribly surprising, then, that a RAND study from 2022 found that subjective social norms were a major influence on people's decision to get the vaccine. People who had a sense that more of their peers were getting the vaccine were more likely to report strong intention to get the vaccine themselves.[54] This finding makes it clear that focusing so heavily on a perceived high level of hesitancy in the Black and Latinx communities might be making the problem worse.

In the conclusion to *Medical Apartheid*, Washington comments on a conflict in Black attitudes toward medicine—a simultaneous need for Black people to enroll in medical research trials in higher numbers to improve the health disparities we see in this country, and a need for Black people to be wary of this research all the same.[8(p388)] And yet, somewhat counterintuitively, Washington argues that "acknowledging abuse and encouraging African Americans to participate in medical research are compatible goals."[8(p388)] This simultaneous encouragement of greater access to healthcare and participation in medical research and recognition of all the myriad reasons why both Black and Latinx communities might be mistrustful are absolutely essential.

In this chapter, I have tried to paint a much more complex and nuanced picture of medical mistrust in these communities, in much the same way I did in the first chapter on the general population. COVID-19 has only increased this sense of ambivalent trust across a variety of sub-populations in the United States. Our only hope at improving the relationship of the general populace with the healthcare system is first and foremost to acknowledge this ambivalence. I have also shown how seemingly everyday, "mundane" problems like access to healthcare have a major influence on trust. This is true for all populations in the United States. Now that I have spent some time looking at mistrust in various formulations, in the next chapter I will explore the more sinister relative of mistrust: conspiracy theories.

3

The Unbearable Mundaneness
of Conspiracy Theories

"Tell me about the person or people that made you want to talk
to me about conspiracy theories and medical mistrust."—Dr. Sara
Gorman, interviewer
           "Half my family."—nearly every interviewee (2022–2023)

Intimately tied to the twin notions of mistrust and distrust is the conspiracy
theory. Conspiracy theories may be a consequence of extreme feelings of
mistrust and distrust. In the world of health and medicine, this means that
people who are prone to mistrust the healthcare system can also be prone
to believing outlandish theories about doctors and health officials. In this
chapter, I will give a little background into the traditional structure of conspiracy theories and argue that the modern conspiracy theory is something different from that traditional model. I will show how conservative
politicians and media have co-opted conspiracy theories and made them
function in "sound bites" that make them easier to pick up on. In other words,
conspiracy theories have been forced into the mainstream, so while we may
not see an increase in the number of people believing in full-blown conspiracy theories, we see a greater portion of the American public believing
in general, more diluted conspiratorial thinking. In addition, thanks largely
to social media, I would describe these new "bite size" conspiracy theories as
decentralized. They often do not have a charismatic leader at the helm and
are more pliable for individuals to shape them in ways that best fit into their
preexisting belief system. This again makes it easier to adopt some version of
conspiratorial thinking on a much broader scale than we have seen before.
These bite-size versions of conspiracy theories used by mainstream political
and media figures as talking points have created a situation in which people
who would normally be "on the fence" get pulled into believing conspiracy

theories. It is these people, the so-called movable middle, who must be reached with the utmost urgency.

This new structure of conspiracy theories as being smaller, more mainstream ideas may partly explain why during my interviews, I regularly heard phrases like "he seemed so logical" or "she seemed so rational otherwise," among others. In these cases, people had not embraced full-blown conspiracy theories but were engaging with some version of different conspiratorial thoughts. These conspiratorial thoughts were often fed to them by conservative politicians and the media. The profile was almost never of someone who was particularly paranoid or irrational. It rather looked as though they had been pulled into somewhat of a slippery slope toward conspiratorial thinking that started with a few stray conspiratorial thoughts. We will come back to this, but first a brief history of conspiracy theories and scholarly thinking about their nature and spread, as well as how this has evolved over time.

The History and Nature of General and Medical Conspiracy Theories

Conspiracy theories are not a new phenomenon. The first record of a medical conspiracy theory can be traced back to 331 BCE, when a plague was killing the citizens of ancient Rome. In this scenario, according to ancient Roman historical sources, some proposed that there was a ring of women who were creating poisons to infect people, and that these poisons represented the origin of the plague.[1] After the great fires in Rome in the year 64 CE, Tacitus, an ancient Roman writer and historian, wrote about rumors that gangs of thugs kept citizens from fighting the fires and that the corrupt emperor Nero had set the devastating fire for his own aims.[2(p87)] During the 14th century, many Europeans believed that Jews were poisoning the wells, which led to Bubonic plague.[1] Conspiracy theories have been especially popular during times of political upheaval. In the aftermath of the French Revolution, many citizens of France attributed events that transpired as the machinations of secret societies such as the Freemasons or the Bavarian Illuminati. After the Russian Revolution, the idea of an international Judeo-Bolshevik conspiracy appealed to many in Europe and North America and finally made its way to the United States early in the Cold War.[3]

Conspiracy theories have been prevalent throughout much of human history but have taken different forms at different points in time. The scholarly understanding of conspiracy theories has also changed over time. In 1945, in his book *The Open Society and Its Enemies*, Karl Popper, who was generally considered one of the greatest philosophers of science of the 20th century, offered a somewhat dismissive definition of conspiracy theories that differs from current approaches to the term and concept. For Popper, conspiracy theories were primarily false and dangerous ideas that spread throughout the population.

In 2004, Bruno Latour, a philosopher, anthropologist, and sociologist, revisited Popper's definition and added the notion of conspiracy theories as social critique. With Latour's definition, we begin to get a better sense of the ways that conspiracy theories mirror contemporary societal preoccupations.[4] In the modern era, Theodor Adorno and Richard Hofstadter have even argued that conspiracy theories and the paranoia that accompanies them are central ingredients of most political movements.[5] This viewpoint suggests that conspiracy theories are quite important and central in moments of political and social change and unrest, rather than being seen as fringe notions that affect only those who are somewhat deranged. Along these lines, multiple interviewees shared with me that their family members' conspiracy theorizing started or worsened during the pandemic. One of them discussed how his father always flirted with conspiracy theories, but his real engagement with them ballooned during the pandemic. Another told me that her mother became more seriously entrenched in other conspiracy theories and more isolated when the COVID vaccines came out and she had concerns. In these common cases, we are seeing a response to a moment of social upheaval in the form of belief in conspiracy theories.

There are several, sometimes competing, ways that people try to conceptualize conspiracy theories. Some have focused on personal characteristics that make certain individuals more prone to falling for conspiracy theories. Efforts to put conspiracy theories into political, social, and historical context are often more convincing than a singular focus on the characteristics of individual people who believe in conspiracy theories. The French philosopher and anthropologist Didier Fassin has argued that purely cognitive accounts of conspiracy theories (e.g., those that focus exclusively on who believes conspiracy theories and who does not) fail to help us understand why conspiracy theories spread more vigorously during certain times and in certain places.[4]

It is this phenomenon that requires sociological and historical explanations. It is especially important to note the close connection between conspiracy theories and politics. It is common for people who maintain medical conspiracy theories to also maintain political conspiracy theories and vice versa. Sometimes the two are so entangled, it is difficult to tell them apart. Many political conspiracy theories contain medical conspiracist beliefs.[6] These medical conspiracy theories are associated with actual changes in health behavior.[7] As Fassin notes, conspiracy theories reveal a double crisis—a crisis of truth *and* a crisis of authority. Conspiracy theories not only question the direct truth of certain accounts, but represent a social critique that questions the authority of society's predominant voices.[4] A conspiracy theory operates as an alternative explanation of an official account.[4] Indeed, distrust of "officialdom" is often a moderating force between conspiracy theories and pure political ideology.[8] Conspiracy theories are often thought of as containing two core beliefs: (1) epistemic mistrust, a fundamental mistrust of conventional, "authoritative" knowledge; and (2) biased information processing and exposure to misinformation, which is often determined by a person's social networks, these days increasingly online.[9]

Where do conspiracy theories come from? I often get the question of whether I think everyone who believes in conspiracy theories is delusional. This seems to me epidemiologically impossible, given the difference between the percentage of people in the population who have psychotic disorders such as schizophrenia (around 1%)[10] and the percentage of people in the population who believe in at least one conspiracy theory (around 50%).[11] One key distinction is that conspiracy theories are a shared social phenomenon, while delusions tend to be private notions espoused by individuals. Delusional content tends to be self-contained and subjective, while conspiracy theories seek to help groups of people make sense of the world around them and unite over a common belief.[12]

Turning our attention now more fully to medical conspiracy theories, it's important to note that they are surprisingly pervasive in our modern world. A nationally representative survey of the U.S. population asked if people agreed with the following statement: "The Food and Drug Administration is deliberately preventing the public from getting natural cures for cancer and other diseases because of pressure from drug companies"; 37% agreed, 31% were unsure, and only 32% actually disagreed.[13(p16)] These kinds of viewpoints are similarly prevalent in underserved communities: in a survey of 500 Black participants, for example, 37.4% agreed that "[m]edical and public health institutions use poor and minority people as guinea pigs to try out new birth control methods," and 24.8% agreed that "[p]oor and minority women are sometimes forced to be sterilized by the government."[13(p60)] Belief in health-related conspiracy theories in particular is often exacerbated whenever there's a health crisis, such as the COVID-19 pandemic. Howard Markel, a medical historian, has called misinformation and conspiracy theories the "lifeblood" of epidemics. During the Zika epidemic in Latin America in 2015–2016, the Annenberg Public Policy Center at the University of Pennsylvania found that 19% of more than 1,000 Americans said they believed microcephaly could result when pregnant women drank water containing pesticides used to fend off mosquitoes.[14] Of course, medical conspiracy theories have been rampant in the wake of COVID-19. As of 2020, at least 25% of the American population reported some level of belief in the idea that the COVID-19 pandemic was somehow planned by malicious actors.[15] In recent years, roughly one in five Americans have said they know someone who believes in QAnon, a mostly online web of conspiracy theories that, among other things, purports that Democratic members of the government and Hollywood are engaged in a large, underground pedophilic ring.[16] This particular network of conspiracy theories gained traction during the COVID-19 pandemic.

It is worth taking a closer look at some of the ideas espoused by conspiracy theorists at various points in medical history to get a better sense of how broad their nature can be, spanning many topics and beliefs in secret, organized activity by some bad actor. I will take one example from the chronic Lyme disease community and one more recent example from the COVID pandemic. First, a little background on chronic Lyme. Lyme disease is a tickborne disease caused by the bacteria *Borrelia burgdorferi*. It is usually successfully treated by a course of antibiotics. Some patients, many of whom have no clinical evidence of current or past infection with *B. burgdorferi*, assert they have long-term symptoms from a past Lyme infection, most commonly fatigue, joint and muscle pain, and brain fog. Because of the inability to pinpoint any known biological basis for these complaints, many physicians resist the term "chronic Lyme" altogether. This has created a fair amount of tension between the medical community and the chronic Lyme community. Conspiracy theories about Lyme disease have, not surprisingly, arisen in the context of this tension and have diminished trust in the medical community. Some have maintained that the U.S. government accidentally or purposely released a large number of infected ticks into the population. This idea is advanced by one chronic Lyme patient, Kris Newby, in her memoir entitled *Bitten: The Secret History of Lyme Disease and Biological Weapons*. In the following quotation from the end of the book, we see Newby advance an idea that is difficult to support, but also a series of recommendations for public health institutions in the United States that are equally difficult to disagree with:

> What this book brings to light is that the U.S. military has conducted thousands of experiments exploring the use of ticks and tick-borne diseases as biological weapons, and in some cases, these agents escaped into the environment. The government needs to declassify the details of these open-air bioweapons tests so that we can begin to repair the damage these pathogens are inflicting on humans and animals in the ecosystem. Where did this devil's brew of tick-borne diseases come from? If you believe Willy Burgdorfer—and I do—there was a deliberate release or an accident, an experiment with unintended consequences to the environment . . . the only way to know the truth is for a whistleblower to step forward or for a classified report to be released. . . . My hope is that this book will widen the lens on our view of this problem and inspire people to more aggressively pursue solutions. We need the CDC to streamline and bring more accuracy to our tick-borne disease surveillance system. We need more DNA detectives to decode the genomes of these pathogens so we can devise ways to disrupt the damage they do. We need epidemiologists to analyze the ongoing spread of these diseases, incorporating the possibility that they were spread in an unnatural way. We need "big data" medical bioinformaticians to analyze our electronic medical records to define diagnostic symptom profiles that map disease combinations and geographic locations. And finally, we need the next generation of bright, curious scientists to lead the charge.[17(pp249–250)]

While it is difficult to imagine that the U.S. military purposely or even accidentally unleashed tick-borne diseases as a biological weapon, it is easy to agree that the CDC needs to do a better job with surveillance, not just of tick-borne diseases, but of all previously occurring and new pathogens in our midst. Perhaps even more importantly, the CDC needs to do a far better job of communicating with U.S. citizens about emerging threats and putting their risk in context. Better utilizing "big data" is similarly an excellent idea. The point here is that while the conspiracy theory itself is unsupported, the frustrated sentiment deriving from obvious areas in which our public health system is failing us is well-founded.

We can see something similar in a conspiracy-theory-ridden paper by a frustrated doctor, published in early 2022:

> While these attacks on free speech are terrifying enough, even worse is the virtually universal control hospital administrators have exercised over the details of medical care in hospitals. These hirelings are now instructing doctors which treatment protocols they will adhere to and which treatments they will not use, no matter how harmful the "approved" treatments are or how beneficial the "unapproved" treatments are. Never in this history of American medicine have hospital administrators dictated to its physicians how they will practice medicine and what medications they can use. The CDC has no authority to dictate to hospitals or doctors concerning medical treatments. Yet, most physicians complied without the slightest resistance.[18(p167)]

In this passage, the author airs some legitimate grievances about the modern medical system. Administrators have acquired too much power, leaving doctors with diminishing autonomy. The CDC often does a less-than-stellar job at communicating with physicians and other members of the general population about new guidelines and the rationale behind them. It is not uncommon for physicians to feel burdened by new guidelines that demand a change in the way they normally practice. He goes on to talk about the "great reset" that has created a "new world order" at the hands of the "elite": "This new world order has been on the drawing boards of the elite manipulators for over a century." While this kind of sentence is classic conspiracy theory rhetoric, with its focus on a powerful elite group that has manipulated us all into a new way of doing things, he still returns to a logical critique of modern medicine, noting that the medical system has become overly "bureaucratized and regimented."[18(p167)] It's difficult to disagree with this, even if it is surrounded by paranoid thinking.

Conspiracy Theories in the Contemporary World: QAnon and Beyond

Now that we have a sense of what conspiracy theories are, the fact that they contain elements of current social and political truth, and that they have been around for as long as we have, we have to ask: Are contemporary conspiracy theories different? Is there anything about conspiracy theories in the COVID era that's unique?

Before I answer that question (or try to answer that question), it's important to establish what some of these contemporary conspiracy theories are. We've all heard about the 5G COVID conspiracy theory, and most of us have also heard plenty about QAnon in recent years. Many COVID-19 conspiracy theories centered on the origin of the virus, which is not surprising—this is a common trope in many epidemics, especially those involving a novel disease. We also saw this type of conspiracy theory about Lyme disease within the chronic Lyme community—the idea that tick-borne diseases were released as part of a bioweapon experimentation program. Several bioweapon-like theories have circulated about COVID, with some asserting that the disease was released from the Wuhan Institute of Virology accidentally due to incompetence, and others asserting that the disease was released intentionally. Sometimes people maintain these two ideas simultaneously, illustrating the ease with which conspiracy theorists can hold incompatible viewpoints so long as they all advance a conspiratorial worldview.[19(p47)] One study of COVID-19 conspiracy theory posts found three assertions that the virus is a bioweapon, four assertions that the virus's real purpose is to allow for increasing government control over the population, and two essentially anti-Semitic assertions that American and Israeli agents released the virus in China. There was also the theory that the Chinese released the virus in order to cause a pandemic, a reference to the idea that the virus is triggered by radiation from 5G networks, or that the virus was a cover-up for broader installation of 5G towers, and the idea that the vaccine contains a microchip to track citizens.[19(p19)] We can see here the variety of ideas comprising COVID-19 conspiracy theories, which is not surprising. Conspiracy theories have the tendency to expand and elaborate on themselves as they get passed throughout the population.

As far as the content of these conspiracy theories goes, there's not too much that's new here. The bioweapon idea has been around for decades and accompanies many concerns about various infectious diseases. Fear of new technology, and 5G in particular, has been with us for years, so the leap to connecting 5G with COVID is not necessarily surprising. Anti-Semitic and racist tendencies are bound up in many conspiracy theories, and COVID-19 conspiracy theories are no different. And yet, when we dig a little deeper into modern-day conspiracy theories, we *do* see something different. Many contemporary conspiracy theories lack a charismatic leader and are thus open to a greater degree of flexibility and interpretation. This flexibility may attract a wider range of individuals to engage in conspiracy-theory thinking, which might partially explain why these ideas seem so much more prevalent in our society today. There is no better place to observe this phenomenon than in the complex, interwoven set of conspiracy theories that comprise the QAnon movement.

QAnon is best known as a conspiracy theory that posits that a wide range of Democratic figures and Hollywood celebrities have been involved for many years in an underground pedophilia ring and that Trump has been selected to put an end to this abuse in an upcoming act of heroism. While these notions are at the center of the QAnon conspiracy theory, the movement as a whole is actually diffuse and multifaceted. As John Bodner and colleagues have noted, QAnon "didn't make anyone do anything." Instead, it is simply a narrative that people want to participate in. How they conceptualize and adapt this narrative to their current lives and beliefs is up to them.[19(pp201–202)] QAnon is, as Mike Rothschild writes in *The Storm Is Upon Us*:

> a complex web of mythology, conspiracy theories, personal interpretations, and assumptions featuring a vast range of characters, events, symbols, shibboleths, and jargon. It can be understood as a conspiracy theory, for sure, but it also touches on aspects of cultic movements, new religions, Internet scams, and political doctrine. It's impossible to fully explicate every aspect of QAnon because it is so diffuse and has so many different plot strands and meanings.[2(p2)]

The content of QAnon conspiracy theories is nothing new. The obsession with wealthy Jewish bankers such as George Soros, a billionaire investor and philanthropist, is a tale as old as time. The obsession with Soros in particular extends back decades, consisting of lies about his childhood, business dealings, and philanthropy. Similarly, conspiracy theories about the five international financier sons of Mayer Rothschild go back all the way to 1812, and the list of central banks owned by the Rothschilds that Q (QAnon's "leader") posted was taken from an ultra-right-wing website listing from 2013.[2(p50)] Even the adrenochrome myth—the notion that a certain necessary biological substance that keeps the rich alive and wealthy must be taken from live children—is just a version of the ancient blood libel, the notion that Jews feast on the blood of Christian children for sustenance.

While QAnon is a patchwork of unoriginal conspiracy theories, it is actually quite difficult to characterize as a movement. The most important part of this definition is the "personal interpretations." QAnon's "leader" Q (more on that in a moment) rewards these kinds of "personal interpretations," encouraging a kind of dialoguing with his theories as opposed to a more central form of "monologuing" that can be seen as characteristic of most conspiracy theory movements with charismatic leaders at the top of their hierarchies. While QAnon might *sound* like an "end-times" cult, with its focus on a morally corrupt group of leaders of the human race who must be censured and disposed of in a heroic, apocalyptic act, this focus on "dialoguing" really distinguishes QAnon from these types of groups.[2(p2)] Indeed, Rothschild justly concludes that QAnon is in some ways impossible to define because it is so diffuse.[2(p2)]

In conversation with Jan-Willem van Prooijen, a noted conspiracy theory scholar, he shared that he did not believe that QAnon meets the criteria for "conspiracy theory," strictly speaking. It is rather better described as a movement bound together by a broad set of conspiratorial ideas with a common theme. He struggled to pinpoint how to classify it. It is also not clear what the directive is for people who subscribe to it. Most conspiracy theories empower people to play detective and find out the "truth." There is nothing so obvious in the case of QAnon.

This focus on personal interpretations and the fact that Q has now all but disappeared create a situation in which we have a tapestry of conspiracy theories that lack a charismatic leader. As I argued in my book *Denying to the Grave*, it is common for conspiracy theories to originate with a charismatic leader who forms a strong group of followers around him or her and creates a potent sense of "us" versus "them" that can, in its most extreme forms, lead to hatred and violence. This is certainly true of past medical conspiracy theories, such as the idea that childhood vaccines cause autism and that HIV is not the cause of AIDS but rather a radical plot by the government to control the population and that life-saving antiretrovirals are poison. QAnon has evolved to encompass a wide range of medical conspiracy theories, mostly centered around COVID-19, but the combination of the disappearance of Q and the fact that QAnon is a patchwork of people's personal interpretation makes it difficult to define it either as a cult or as a conspiracy theory network headed by a charismatic leader. QAnon cannot strictly be called a cult because there are often long stretches in which Q is silent, and followers end up filling the void with their own directives. This is something no cult leader would normally allow.[2] The result is a free-for-all that often allows people to *think* they are not becoming radicalized because they are definitively not joining a cult or becoming ensnared in the orders of a charismatic leader, and they are simply innocently using Q's ideas as a jumping-off point to express notions they already hold.

This pattern became clear during the pandemic, when more diverse groups of people began engaging with QAnon. QAnon followers were often at the center of COVID-19 conspiracy theories. During the pandemic, new populations were radicalized, including people who hated Donald Trump and wouldn't necessarily associate with right-wing politics.[2(p124)] During the pandemic, isolated, lonely moms were one group of people who began falling for QAnon beliefs. A sub-community called "QA-Mom" arose, which targeted and won over a number of lifestyle influencers. One researcher called this phenomenon "Pastel QAnon" because the rhetoric was "softer" around the edges compared to traditional QAnon followers. Many of the "QA-Mom" followers were left-leaning but anti-vaccine and anti-science and seemed to genuinely believe the QAnon-related content they were sharing.[2(pp128–129)] In my interviews, I heard many casual mentions of QAnon. It was a mainstay of a very diverse group of believers, from California liberals to incarcerated African American men to people who just seemed to go down the rabbit hole by accident.

And then during the summer of 2020 came the "#SaveTheChildren" campaign, which co-opted a hashtag usually used to draw attention to the real international problem of child trafficking, in order to advance the conspiracy theory that an international cabal of elites, including many top political officials in the United States, were involved in a child-trafficking scheme. The "campaign" was momentarily blocked by Facebook. It was broad enough to capture the imaginations of people who might never normally sign on to QAnon rhetoric. The campaign exploded especially on Facebook, where anti-vaccine and anti-trafficking groups saw their followings increase by thousands of percent. As Mike Rothschild notes, "Many of the people coming to Q from anti-trafficking posts through #SaveTheChildren had no idea what Q was or what it meant. Some weren't even Trump supporters. But fueled by pandemic fears and a genuine desire to 'do something,' they radicalized themselves quickly and efficiently."[2(p133)] QAnon's messaging has often been broad and appealing enough to attract large swaths of people, some of whom are not even right-leaning or particularly prone to conspiracy theories under normal circumstances, to espouse its central values of protecting our nation's children and to make QAnon messaging their own. The pandemic, with all its uncertainties and negative social consequences, created a perfect breeding ground for these ideas, in all their variations, to take hold of greater portions of the population.

Then there is, of course, the "gaming" aspect of QAnon, which makes it much like an escape from reality. This is a distinctive element as well—most conspiracy theories are mired in reality as they attempt to explain everything going on around us. QAnon, on the other hand, allows for this escape into a gaming world in which themes from the conspiracy theories are present but the focus is not on uncovering a wide-ranging political scheme. This gaming aspect, most likely unique to the online version of conspiracy theories, also draws in a population of gamers who might otherwise stay away. On the whole, the most significant contemporary version of a conspiracy theory we have is one that allows for broader engagement on the fringes, rather than only attracting people who are die-hard acolytes. So how do we define people who believe in conspiracy theories when this is our new version of what they are?

Who Believes in Conspiracy Theories?

There have been many attempts over the years to "characterize" people who might be more prone to believe in conspiracy theories. Some have speculated that conspiracy theorists are pathologically ill with a form of paranoia or psychosis, but this viewpoint has largely been discredited because conspiracy theories are too widespread to be entirely pathological. As Jan-Willem van Prooijen has argued, they are the domain of social psychology, not clinical psychology.[13(p17)] There have been speculations surrounding trust and group membership, such as the notion that people who are less inclined to trust others in general might be more prone to conspiracy theories.[13(p10)] In addition, stronger identification with a group will increase chances of conspiracy beliefs because people draw stronger contrasts between the ingroup and the outgroup, and because they care more about people in the ingroup being victimized.[13(p53)] The more dissimilar the outgroup, the more likely people are to believe conspiracy theories about them, again heightening the "us versus them" dynamic.[13(p10)] Cassam has argued that people who believe in conspiracy theories often give themselves over to certain "epistemic vices," such as gullibility, wishful thinking, close-mindedness, and prejudice, such that it is not just that they are exposed to poor-quality information, but that it is also absorbed in a particular way by conspiracy-prone individuals.[20(pp113-114)] In a turn that ties together the two themes of this book (mistrust and conspiracy theories), it has often been argued that conspiracy theories are really about distrust of authorities and institutions and a deeply held belief that looks a lot like religion but is not tied to any particular theology.[13(p46)]

Perspective-taking is another feature that can lead to stronger conspiracy beliefs. In one Dutch study, participants read about an opposition leader in Benin who died in a car crash. None of the participants had any particular connection with Benin. In the study, the participants heard about one of two potential consequences of the crash: in one scenario, the opposition leader died and the election was postponed; in the other scenario, the opposition leader survived with just minor bruising. Half of the participants were given perspective-taking instructions, in which they were asked to think about the situation from the viewpoint of the current leader. Then they tried to elicit conspiracy theories about the opposition leader's death. Conspiracy theories were more prominent in the scenario in which the opposition leader died, but only among people who received perspective-taking instructions.[13(p55)] The suggestion here is that there may be a pro-social inkling at the center of conspiracy theory thinking that unfortunately often ends up having an anti-social consequence. This is not entirely surprising: the strong association with one's group is also a pro-social impulse that becomes anti-social when it is used to turn against people who seem different from those in the ingroup.

There is also a tendency to try to understand whether conspiracy theories are more common on one or the other side of the political aisle. Some have argued that people on the political right are more likely to believe in conspiracy theories because they have a stronger preference for order and score higher on a variable called "social dominance orientation," which measures tolerance for inequalities across groups in a society.[13(p66)] At the same time, it seems equally plausible that people on any extreme might be more prone to conspiracy theories, whether they be on the extreme left or the extreme right. People at both ends of the spectrum are more likely to believe in conspiracy theories, mostly those that have to do with collective interests, such as climate change, war, financial crises, and so on. These individuals do not necessarily score higher on measures of everyday paranoia, such as believing that someone is following them.[13(p77)] It is also possible that conspiracy theories are more pronounced among those on the left in countries where the left is more radicalized (like some countries in Latin America), and more pronounced among those on the right in countries where the right is more radicalized (like the U.S. at present).[13(p76)]

In many of my interviews, I could not easily discern a political pattern among the people who were described to me. I heard many examples of people on the extreme left who bought into certain conspiracy theories, mostly about the environment and food sources. I also heard examples of QAnon Trump followers who thought government interference in vaccination was a conspiracy. Many people described relatives who seemed to start off in one political camp and yet eventually espoused conspiratorial beliefs of the other side, often without realizing it.

In a recent conversation with conspiracy theory researcher and political scientist Joseph Uscinski, he shared with me his belief that the Internet and social media have not radicalized people en masse, or in the way many people have argued, and that people who believe in conspiracy theories were likely going to believe in them regardless. His research did not show a notable increase in the portion of the population who believe in conspiracy theories during the COVID-19 pandemic, despite it being a seemingly ripe time for them to perpetuate, given the vast amount of social and political uncertainty and the immediate threat of an increased risk to the population's health and well-being. It is easy to see how some people might become radicalized under such circumstances, perhaps becoming more paranoid about government bodies that make one recommendation one day and reverse it the next, about a disease whose origins were objectively somewhat of a mystery, at least at first. But Uscinski did not see evidence of this, instead arguing that people's thinking "remains stable over time." Indeed, his recent research bears this point out: in a study of letters written to the editors of the *New York Times* and *Chicago Tribune* between 1890 and 2010, Uscinski and his collaborator Joseph Parent did not find a significant increase in conspiracy beliefs over time. Instead, the phenomenon seems to have remained relatively stable.

Not everyone agrees with this perspective. In conversation with Jan-Willem van Prooijen, he shared his belief that conspiracy theories now spread much faster than ever before and it is easier to find like-minded people online. This sense of community makes conspiracy theories more entrenched. In addition, he commented that the use of social media to discuss medical and health topics has reduced people's need to consult experts and has allowed for medical conspiracy theories to spread with greater ease.

If Uscinki's idea that conspiracy theories have remained relatively stable in the midst of the social and political upheaval accompanying the pandemic is correct, then it follows that they must not be caused by external forces but must be more dependent on character traits and predispositions within individuals. This is a common line of inquiry for many conspiracy-theory researchers trying to understand what might make some individuals more prone to conspiracy theories than others. As noted previously, the answer is most likely not pathology. We do already know that people with strong ingroup affinities are more likely to believe in conspiracy theories. What about other factors, such as anxiety, education level, gender, age, and so on? In 2020, a study by Uscinski and collaborators found no association between level of educational attainment and conspiracy beliefs.[21] There is a fair amount of debate on this attribute and its relationship to conspiracy theories, but Uscinski and collaborators maintain that conspiracy theories have more to do with psychological and political affinities and tendencies than with non-psychological factors such as degree of education. Gender has also never seemed to have a strong relationship with conspiracy theories one way or the other, at least not consistently in the literature. In Uscinski's study, factors that were associated with conspiracy theory beliefs were the tendency to reject expert opinions and accounts of major events and a somewhat vague predisposition to view major events as part of a conspiracy theory pattern. Partisan and ideological motivations were also strongly associated with believing in conspiracy theories, especially for people who supported Trump and followed politics closely.[21] So political, ideological, and psychological motivations and tendencies seem to be at the center of conspiracy theory beliefs in this study and in Uscinski's current thinking in general. Yet, while identifying the factors that make individuals more prone to believing conspiracy theories is important, there are larger issues that determine how potent and widespread these theories are. There are unique larger factors at play now, especially during the pandemic, that make some aspects of conspiracy theories different from how they have traditionally operated.

Who believed in conspiracy theories during the COVID-19 pandemic? And what about QAnon? Are these the same people that Uscinski and others are referring to in their research? In some cases, yes, but there is reason to believe that a different cadre of people are now becoming attracted to conspiracy theories. Many of the conspiracy theories about COVID-19 were ultimately about the vaccine, so in some cases COVID-19 vaccine refusal could be a good proxy for belief in conspiracy theories about the pandemic. One 2021 study found that COVID-19 vaccine acceptance was influenced by many of the same factors that marked acceptance of vaccines (real or theoretical) in previous epidemics, including SARS, MERS, and Ebola. These factors usually included efficacy, minor adverse effects, and protection duration.[22] In our research at Critica, we found the same thing—many who were hesitant about the vaccine cited ideas that the vaccine doesn't work, that it forces you to continue wearing a mask anyway, that it has a lot of side effects, and that its protection wears off quickly. At the same time, the COVID-19 pandemic was accompanied by a lot of factors that could increase mistrust of science and make conspiracy thinking worse. The vaccine was developed on an accelerated schedule, and there was (and still is) a great deal of medical uncertainty about the disease itself. Undermining people's trust in the institutions that deliver healthcare often leads to decreased willingness to engage in preventive health behaviors, such as taking a vaccine.[22] Decreased trust in both science and institutional policymakers can also make people more prone to believe in conspiracy theories.

Some people told me stories that showcased people who were always prone to conspiracy theories. When the pandemic started, they simply jumped on the bandwagon. These people were more likely to believe outlandish ideas like the 5G COVID conspiracy theory or the microchip notion. Everyone I spoke to said COVID made their family members' conspiratorial thinking worse. But equally numerous were those who said belief in full-blown conspiracy theories did not occur until the pandemic. Many were at a loss, as they often described their loved ones as previously completely rational and in many cases pro-science. Most of them started with a shadow of a doubt about the vaccines, but by the time I spoke to their relatives, they fully embraced ideas about COVID as a government conspiracy. It is hard to justify that idea that circumstances surrounding COVID did not impact conspiratorial thinking.

Uscinski and colleagues found that COVID-19 conspiracy theories were tied to a number of personal factors: denialism, partisanship, ideology, religiosity, and youth.[21] Factors such as denialism, religiosity, and youth are commonly found to be associated with conspiracy theory thinking in prior research.[23] Ideology and especially partisanship may be tied to our particular political moment. While strong feelings about ingroups and outgroups are commonly associated with conspiracy thinking, this focus on partisan ideology and the polarization between political parties in the United States has pulled a wide swath of people, especially on the political right, into conspiracy thinking. This has a lot to do with the precise way in which the right-wing media and politicians position themselves.

What about QAnon? Who believes in that? The movement certainly appealed directly to an extremist group of neo-Nazis and fascists, whose exposure to a variety of social media campaigns and their increasing social isolation from family encouraged a kind of mistrust that had "sealed some of these people into a closed propaganda bubble for years." They were essentially waiting in the wings until they were finally "offered an irresistible image of themselves as righteous heroes in a holy war."[24(p359)] Neo-Nazis, neo-fascists, and White supremacists had been sidelined from mainstream political conversation for a long time and were finally able to build up their numbers and following through an association with this new conspiracy theory.[24(p359)] But lest we write QAnon off as a fringe belief, it is important to remember that 55% of Republicans claimed to believe at least a portion of QAnon ideas as of September 2020.[24(p360)]

Amelia Jamison and colleagues had one of the more important findings about online conspiracy theory networks during the COVID-19 pandemic. As she concludes in a 2020 paper: "Online communities are not homogenous; our findings suggest online rumors tend to circulate within smaller subgroups. While many topics overlap, specific arguments are likely to vary. This suggests that a one-size-fits-all approach to combating misinformation is unlikely to work on both vaccine-oriented vaccine opponents and vaccine opponents that are motivated by conservative politics."[25(p4)] Her notion that a "one-size-fits-all" approach to combating misinformation might be inappropriate due to the heterogeneous nature of people who engage with misinformation and conspiracy theories should also make us take pause about such an approach when it comes to defining who exactly becomes convinced of conspiracy theories as well. This is not an uncommon criticism of the "dispositional" approach that tries to define what characteristics determine someone's beliefs in conspiracy theories. For example, it has been argued that the idea that those who feel powerless embrace conspiracy theories is not useful:

> Researchers must learn why people feel this way. Often, it is because of mistreatment by other people or institutions. Women who have experienced oppressive reproductive regimes, such as that in Romania during the regime of Nicolae Ceasescu, frequently opt out of immunization. People who get vaccinated generally do so not because of an understanding of immunology, but because of trust in—and access to—health-care systems.[26(p765)]

In other words, there are cultural and historical factors that determine acceptance of science and belief in conspiracy theories.

Another account based on work by the anthropologist Elisa Sobo points out that even when conspiracy theories sound similar in content, their cultural reasoning might differ. For example, in the United States, conspiratorial attacks are usually aimed at certain individuals' "self-built prosperity." In Poland, they centered around the notion that the state was hiding its failures. In Ireland, they often have to do with post-colonial fears of British rule and suspicion surrounding foreign influence.[26] This is how conspiracy theories gain traction—by resonating with relevant local histories, culture, and shared fears. Combating medical conspiracies therefore requires being aware of these unique histories in order to devise counterarguments that will also resonate with the very nature of the fear that people are expressing.[26] For this reason, it might be counterproductive to create personality profiles of people who believe in conspiracy theories because it gets in the way of looking more closely at the system that pushes people toward conspiracy beliefs.[26]

The anthropologist Didier Fassin has argued for different lenses through which to view conspiracy theories. In his view, psychological interpretations of the type I have been outlining do not tell the whole story. These interpretations focus on individual characteristics that may make someone more prone to believing in conspiracy theories, but they cannot explain why larger segments of the population become enamored of these beliefs. In his view, cultural interpretations of the type I have just outlined regarding Ireland, the United States, and Poland, are more sophisticated, but they do not on their own account for why some people are more prone to conspiracy theories than others. Political interpretations usually focus on historically marginalized groups and explore how and why they are prone to conspiracy theories. The best approach is probably to combine these approaches in a method that attempts to understand the various levels on which conspiracy theories take place. This will be an approach I will try to emulate in the remainder of this chapter.

So who *does* believe in conspiracy theories? And is there any reason to believe that this population is different now from what it was 10 or 15 years ago? There are a couple of common traits about conspiracy theorists. One is that they tend to be incredibly moralizing. Their moral righteousness and their sense of their own heroism, which might comprise an element of grandiosity, are often at the center of conspiracy theories. In the book *American Conspiracies and Cover-Ups*, Douglas Cirignano demonstrates this often. For example, in espousing a common myth that AIDS is a plot by the government to reduce the population, he says: "Could AIDS be an official depopulation program, a genocide aimed at two segments of society that have been traditionally ostracized and hated: homosexuals and blacks?"[27(p174)] This focus on the segments of society that have been "traditionally ostracized" gives the statement a moralizing focus, since Cirignano chastises the government for taking aim at groups that are already discriminated against and marginalized. Cirignano employs a similar turn of phrase when discussing the hepatitis B vaccine, which he believes has been contaminated with the AIDS virus: "To some researchers it is time for the government to make another apology, and to admit that the hepatitis B vaccine was contaminated with AIDS and was the cause of America's AIDS epidemic."[27(p171)] Again, his tone is one of moral righteousness. The government needs to "admit" and "make [an] apology." When conspiracy theorists ask a powerful body to come clean about the supposed plot they are covering up, the demand is normally shrouded in confessional language that seems more a matter of morals and ethics than anything else. Conspiracy theorists often believe that they are the center of the very battle between Good and Evil.

In her memoir about her journey with an alleged case of chronic Lyme, Kris Newby talks about her experience with uncovering the supposed conspiracy at the center of increasing cases of Lyme in the United States as if it is a moral calling:

> Grey had sent me the video because he wanted my help with his investigation. I hesitated. I had battled Lyme disease for seven years and had been symptom-free for three, and while I was recovering, I had spent three and a half years working on the Lyme disease documentary. Now I wanted to move on. I had a great job writing about the latest advances in medical research at Stanford University. My kids were almost finished with college. Let someone else carry this torch. I needed boring, safe normalcy. Still, I felt a nagging guilt that the documentary had missed its mark. And if Willy's claim was true, a crime against humanity had been committed by the U.S. government, and then covered up. If the full story weren't told, millions more Lyme patients would suffer. Somebody needed to dig out the truth, and I figured that somebody was me.[17(p101)]

In this illustrative passage, Newby discusses her choice as one clouded by ambivalence. She details how she wants to just live a quiet life with her "great job" and her children. And yet something was calling her, producing a sense of "nagging guilt." Her realization that she needs to continue working on this is dramatic: "Somebody needed to dig out the truth, and I figured that somebody was me." Her mission is no less than to save "millions more Lyme patients" from needless suffering. Her dramatic tale of her own struggle with the conspiracy and her realization that she was compelled by her sense of moral duty to uncover it plays right into the hands of most conspiracy theory narratives. Those who work to uncover them are morally superior, ethical models of all that is right in the world, in a battle against the evil oppressor. It would not be too far off the mark to describe them as selfless martyrs, as many historical martyrs were involved in battles against the establishment. Newby's hesitation could even be said to be reminiscent of something like St. Augustine's 4th-century ambivalence in his *Confessions*, in the scene in the garden in which he struggles and finally takes up the Bible and reads and is converted. This sudden realization of the greatness of God is similar in its sense of moral duty and righteousness to Newby's sudden realization of her calling to uncover the grave injustice that the U.S. government has wrought on its innocent victims. This pattern of moralizing represents a major feature of the largest contemporary conspiracy theory: QAnon. It is a hallmark of QAnon to believe that one is in a righteous battle against the evil Democrats, who are literally abusing children, in this movement's view.

Conspiracy theorists aren't always extremists, though. The non-extremist flavor of conspiracy theories has been especially true throughout the pandemic. But even before COVID, we see some conspiracy theorists approach their own beliefs with a certain amount of subtlety and caution. In her memoir *Bitten*, Newby describes her realization that, in her view, Lyme disease was not naturally occurring, but rather a pathogen released by the U.S. government as part of a secret bioweapons program:

> It was a stunning admission from one of the world's foremost authorities on Lyme disease. If it was true, it meant that Willy had left out essential data from his scientific articles on the Lyme disease outbreak, and that as the disease spread like a wildfire in the Northeast and Great Lakes regions of the United States, he was part of the cover-up of the truth. He seemed to be saying that Lyme wasn't a naturally occurring germ, one that may have gotten loose and been spread by global warming, an explosion of deer, and other environmental changes. It had been created in a military bioweapons lab for the specific purpose of harming human beings. And somehow it had gotten out.[17(p99)]

Even at the height of her conviction about this supposedly massive cover-up, Newby is circumspect about how the pathogen escaped the lab. "Somehow it had gotten out," she says. We would perhaps expect her to be more forward at this point, blaming the American scientists for perhaps purposely leaking pathogens into the general population and then covering it up with gusto. That would probably be our expectation given what we know about conspiracy theories from media coverage and the literature—that they are extreme. However, it is clear that Newby is not certain that this is what happened, and she is not shy about admitting that. In her account, it is not a threat to her beliefs that she is not sure about every detail or the motive behind the release of the pathogens, if there was one. While her ideas may be seen as generally strong and, in some cases, extreme, she does not present herself as the all-out extremist we might expect.

This view of conspiracy theorists as not necessarily "all-out extremists" has also emerged throughout the pandemic. People who were previously "on board" with science seemed to fall into bizarre beliefs out of nowhere. There was a poignant story covered by NPR in April 2022 about an older woman who seemed to fit this description. Her family sometimes teased her for being interested in astrology and spirituality, but she was always a strong advocate for science-based health interventions such as vaccines. Her husband recalled lovingly: "She made sure I took the flu shots, we took the shingles shot, we took the pneumonia shot. . . . I mean, I was like a pincushion." But when the pandemic started, she began watching an increasing number of concerning videos. The videos told her that the pandemic was a hoax. She had a spiritual group that met at her house weekly and none of her compatriots believed the pandemic was real either. Her husband called it "tribal" and worried that the members of the group were reinforcing each other's faulty beliefs. She eventually subscribed to the belief that the COVID vaccines had microchips in them that would allow Bill Gates and the government to track her movements. She also believed that the vaccines were somehow being used to spread the disease. As a result, despite her perfect vaccination track record, she refused to get vaccinated against COVID.[28] She eventually died of COVID, after a hospital stay in which she refused all the available treatments. Her husband, who was in the hospital at the same time and accepted all treatments offered to him, survived. In reflecting on her mother's death, one of Stephanie's daughters said she saw her mother as a victim of online attention-seekers who generate hours of false content each day. As she put it: "Whoever is creating all this content, is on some level waging a war—here in America—inside of every family. . . . I think people need to wake up to that."

In our work at Critica and through interviews conducted for this book, I have now heard from hundreds of people about their conspiratorial beliefs about COVID-19 and the vaccines against it. In our Critica interventions on-line to combat misinformation, we have heard from people in both English and Spanish about their concerns over the vaccine. Many people casually slipped into conspiracy theory beliefs, sometimes seemingly out of no-where. These concerns were very often accompanied by appeals to sources they deemed authorities on the subject. In February 2021, one respondent on Facebook quoted at length from a supposedly authoritative doctor who raised questions about the mRNA vaccines and even cited a quotation from Dr. Peter Hotez, a prominent pediatrician and virologist, saying he did not think the vaccines were ready for primetime (a quote that was taken out of context). This poster also includes the credentials and affiliations of all of his or her "authorities," so that the post read like a who's who of infec-tious disease experts. Other posters appeal to authority by relying heavily on numbers. Even though in many cases these numbers are incorrect or the calculations derived from them are suspect, the point here is that the poster goes through the trouble of laying out his or her reasoning by walking us through a series of calculations that ultimately "prove" that COVID is not a serious illness and that the vaccines are not effective. These appeals to seem-ingly traditional authorities, even if they turn out not to be real authorities or the careful calculations turn out not to be correct, demonstrate how con-spiracy thinking can actually be, or at least start out, mainstream. Posters switch between this rational impulse to trust authority figures into stating more outlandish, conspiracy-laden thinking seamlessly. The leap from the mainstream to the conspiracy is not actually that far in these people's minds. Switching back and forth between these two modes, these posters demon-strate a key feature of the 21st-century and especially the COVID-era con-spiracy theory: that it is in many ways more strongly grounded in an inkling of reality than many prior conspiracy theories and that its believers are closer to normal, mainstream thinkers than we might think when we ponder con-spiracy theorists.

Over and over in my interviews, I encountered people who described their family members as hardened conspiracy theorists, while in the same breath saying that they frequently wavered. One person told me his father had a heart attack and refused to go on a statin due to various medical conspiracy theory beliefs. At the same time, he told me that his father's mother often had the capacity to make him reconsider. Numerous others detailed family members' entrenched conspiracy theories, but then also told me that those same family members got vaccinated against COVID after some pressure from family members.

When it comes to the pandemic, some of the most common conspiracy theories have a mundane undertone to them. While more outlandish conspiracy theories exist—for example, about the supposed microchip Bill Gates placed in the vaccine to track people, or the idea that 5G technology was responsible for creating a pandemic in order to divert people's attention from a hostile takeover of society—these ideas are not that prevalent in the population. Instead, we find a lot more doubt, fear, and suspicion surrounding the vaccine and official statistics and statements about the nature of the virus. People with conspiracy beliefs about the pandemic commonly purport one or all of several notions: (1) that the COVID death rate has been inflated by doctors who want to make more money from insurance claims; (2) that the mRNA vaccines pose dangers that are being kept from the public by the pharmaceutical companies and the government as part of a profit motive; and (3) that there was some outright misconduct involved in the vaccine trials that may have skewed the results. There is also the less commonly held belief that the virus escaped from a lab in Wuhan and that the U.S. government knew this all along but has been lying to protect the profits they have reaped from certain forms of research around the globe. Very few people seem to subscribe to the theory that the virus was released intentionally by the Chinese, although the idea is occasionally out there. These notions, while bizarre and full of misinformation, do not quite rise to the level of the idea that Lyme disease is the result of an elaborate, purposeful release of pathogens into the American public by way of a secret U.S. bioweapons program that cannot be confirmed to even exist in the first place. There is much less machination and assumption of pure evil in the kinds of conspiracy theories that have accompanied COVID. They are more purely the kinds of thoughts and ideas that arise from a truly fearful, weary, and suspicious population. These ideas smack of uncertainty and fatigue after several years of following government directives that have not always been well communicated. They are not, on the face of it, on par with the most extreme forms of conspiracy theories we have seen throughout the 20th and early 21st centuries.

In interviews I conducted in 2022 and 2023, I found much the same thing. Many people who were currently espousing conspiratorial beliefs about COVID told me that prior to the pandemic, they were accepting of sanctioned preventive interventions such as childhood vaccines and that they accepted most or all of what their doctors told them to do. One individual, a business owner located in New York City, told me that he was never suspicious of public health organizations such as the CDC and the FDA before the pandemic. But he started getting frustrated early in the pandemic because he thought the reaction to it was an overreaction. He was especially upset about the restrictions on children, including mandatory virtual school. He called masking children a form of "abuse." He told me he was angry at the FDA and the CDC (and other similar organizations) and no longer trusted them because he believed they were wrong from the beginning, especially in their recommended restrictions on children, when he believed that only old and unwell people were getting that sick with COVID. When I asked him why he thought the government was making recommendations that he deemed "unscientific," he told me that while he did think they were hiding something from the public, he shared: "I don't know why, I don't think it's malicious." Throughout all of this, he maintained the belief that there was nothing suspicious about non-COVID vaccines and that his child was fully vaccinated and would continue to be so, but that he would not be receiving the COVID vaccine. This person shared that he had many left-leaning friends who do not agree with him and that he tried to read balanced sources on political topics, including the *Washington Post*, *New York Times*, *MSNBC*, and *Fox*. He was not on social media. He claimed never to have believed in conspiracy theories before COVID but admitted to being naturally "anti-authoritarian."

Despite the seeming "mildness" of his ideas about COVID, this man subscribed to several popular right-leaning conspiracy theories. For example, he was convinced that the virus came from a lab, not from a meat market in Wuhan, and that the United States was funding "gain of function" research in Wuhan and they didn't want the U.S. public to know about that, so they covered up the whole origin story of the virus, which they knew all along. He claimed there were even emails condemning U.S. officials who knew that virus research at Wuhan Institute of Virology was potentially dangerous and had called for it to be "shut down" but that no one did anything. As we will see, this line of thinking comes straight from right-wing media pundits such as Tucker Carlson and is a classic conspiracy theory in its assertion of a dangerous secret with serious consequences being kept from the public in order to protect the interests and reputation of the government. He believed that the polarization of the media, especially the way the left-wing media treats right-wing political ideas, was partially responsible for some of the cover-up of stories such as the origin of COVID-19. The cover-up was once again not necessarily caused by malice on the part of any identifiable individual or group, but had more to do with the general partisanship that is rampant today. While this man certainly espoused several real conspiracy theories around COVID and harbored an accompanying deep mistrust of the medical and public health establishment, he may not fit the bill of the type of conspiracist that we see described in the literature on this phenomenon, in part because he was far from being a lifelong conspiracy theory believer. His story is representative of what I've seen of conspiracy theorists surrounding the pandemic through hundreds of interventions and interviews.

One more slightly different example should help solidify the picture of the 21st-century American conspiracist, this time through the eyes of a close relative. One man, a Peruvian-American pharmaceutical company executive, talked to me about two close relatives, mainly a cousin and a brother, who had fallen into several conspiracy theory beliefs, including some notions from QAnon. As he described it, these relatives were always anti-vaxxers but they were both apolitical before Trump. They became Trump supporters during the lead-up to the 2016 election and began repeating whatever Sean Hannity and Tucker Carlson said verbatim shortly after that. Their belief in COVID-19-related conspiracy theories took off as soon as Trump discredited the virus as a serious threat. In this man's view, his relatives felt too ashamed to ever admit they might be wrong and so he felt they were "shoehorning" reality to fit their worldview. He felt that they lived in echo chambers on social media and experienced a lot of confirmation bias in those online contexts. He noted that these were family members with the least amount of education, and he felt they were searching for certainty in their lives. He described both his cousin and his brother as feeling as though they had gotten "the short end of the stick" in life—both were blue-collar workers and his cousin was a war veteran, and they both had difficulty finding and keeping jobs. Trump's many proclamations that immigrants were stealing American jobs had great appeal for both of them.

Interestingly, he noted a third family member, a sister-in-law, who was not pro-Trump but was rabidly anti-vaccine (despite being a nurse). She believed that all COVID vaccines were attenuated virus vaccines (which many are not—some are mRNA vaccines, which is a different technology) and that you could get infected from the vaccine (a classic anti-vaxxer argument about attenuated and live virus vaccines that is also not true). She also espoused many QAnon conspiracy beliefs, despite again not being particularly right-wing or a Trump supporter. A lot of her talking points came from fringe, extremist right-wing pundits, but it seemed she often did not realize this was where her ideas were coming from. How do people who seem relatively non-extreme come to be convinced of conspiracy theories? A lot of the answer has to do with the new formulation of modern conspiracy theories such as QAnon, where it truly is "choose your own adventure." Without a charismatic leader controlling the message at all times, people are free to take pieces of what they like about QAnon and disregard the rest. They can believe parts of it but distance themselves from other parts that seem too extreme or that threaten their identity. For example, if they are not pro-Trump, they can still espouse QAnon beliefs without subscribing to the notion that it is Trump who will be our salvation and save us from corrupt liberal pedophiles and criminals. It turns out that much of the political and media rhetoric on the right has also operated this way over the past several years, feeding the public bits and pieces of conspiracy theories shrouded in more mild-sounding rhetoric.

"On the Other Hand . . .": Conspiracy Theories "Lite" in the Media and on the Political Stage

Commenting on how an extremist view like replacement theory has become mainstream in right-wing parlance, Jonathan Greenblatt, CEO of the Anti-Defamation League, has traced a straight line from the dark web to Tucker Carlson and Laura Ingraham's talking points on primetime *Fox News*. In his view, ideas that originate on White supremacist message boards or the dark web jump to more mainstream online message boards such as 4chan and 8chan, then to specialty "news" sources such as Breitbart and the Daily Caller, and finally to mainstream right-wing media such as Carlson's wildly popular *Fox News* show.[29] When someone like Carlson talks about the great replacement theory, he does not outright say that a "Jewish cabal" is plotting to import immigrants into America in order to replace Americans. As Greenblatt rightly points out, he utilizes language that is more "palatable" for most Americans. He moves away from terms such as "White genocide" in order to attract more Americans to these extremist notions. Greenblatt says they have "repackaged" the ideas to make them look like political partisan issues and that "[i]t has been an intentional effort . . . to take these ideas and to try to sanitize them . . . so they could bring their ideas into the mainstream."

Nowhere is this more at work than in Carlson's show. After analyzing numerous clips from *Tucker Carlson Tonight*, it became obvious to me that the show's conspiracy theory-laden monologues seem to always follow a specific arc. Carlson draws the listener in by appealing to science and seeming not to have too much animosity for the "other side," but then somewhere toward the middle, he turns everything upside down, often using phrases such as "on the other hand" to signal the start of a descent into what often ends up being some serious conspiracy theorizing.

Let's take a few examples to show how prevalent this structure is. In a June 2021 clip in which Carlson ultimately shares conspiracy thinking about the origins of COVID-19, he begins building his case by appealing to authoritative sources such as CNN, *The Lancet,* and Robert Redfield, the former director of the CDC. Of Redfield, whom he purports espouses the notion that the virus leaked from a lab in Wuhan, he even says, "This isn't some guy on Twitter. That's the former director of the CDC." He even has a somewhat sympathetic story about a journalist from another left-leaning media source, the *BBC*, whom he says was thwarted from covering the origins of the virus by the Chinese. He works up to his "punch line" slowly, littering his path with references to authoritative scientific sources and media sources from his rivals to make him look more moderate and rational. Finally, at around nine minutes, he starts to entertain the notion that the Chinese knew about the leak but covered it up, and only toward the end of the clip does he begin to entertain the notion that "some" Americans believe that the U.S. government might have known and covered up the leak as well. The height of the conspiracy theory here is the notion that the U.S. government was in on an intentional leaking of the virus from Wuhan and has been lying to the American public ever since. The idea that a big, powerful entity such as the U.S. government is harboring such a significant lie is classic conspiracy theorizing and one of the central conspiracy theories that has surrounded the pandemic in the United States. But we see how Carlson doesn't get there immediately. While many conspiracy theorists and conspiracy-theory charismatic leaders would come out with these ideas more quickly, Carlson presents a kind of deconstructed, diluted conspiracy theory and works hard to draw his audience in before appealing to their fear and confusion.

Another clip from April 2020 in which Carlson disputes the reported death rate of COVID-19 shows a similar tactic. He once again begins by appealing to authoritative sources, including a Columbia University Medical Center study on COVID-19 rates and outcomes among pregnant women and a guest who is a Stanford University professor of medicine. He even critiques the study in a way that might somewhat refute his ultimate point that the severity and death rate of the virus have been inflated by politicians and government authorities: "215 people is a small sample, and in this particular case, it is not a representative sample. Hospitals are major vectors for the transmission of coronavirus. Pregnant women tend to spend a lot of time in hospitals. Pregnant women are also younger and healthier than most people, so it's possible they're also less likely to exhibit symptoms of the virus." In this quote, he entertains some of the reasons the "opposition" might provide for why the study he's citing does not prove that the virus is not that severe. Once again, toward the middle of the segment, Carlson turns everything on its head by professing "on the other hand": "Meanwhile in Germany, the official death rate from the coronavirus stands today at about 2.5%. That's a horrifying number, and it may be real. On the other hand, in the town of Gangelt, where large-scale testing has been performed, the death rate was found to be just 0.37%. That's a fraction of the official number, it's barely one-seventh of it." Here he begins to float his primary suggestion that the death rate associated with COVID-19 has been wildly inaccurate as reported to the American public. But he doesn't stop there. By the end of the segment, he suggests that the "authorities" might be inflating the death rate and lying to the American public on purpose:

> Above all, if this is true, it would mean that the rest of us could be slightly less terrified going forward . . . it would not quite be the plague we thought it was, and that might give us some perspective. We could begin maybe to think clearly again. Most of us want all of that badly, but do our leaders want that? Sometimes when you watch them you begin to suspect that they're secretly enjoying our fear.

Once again, he works up to this very slowly and does not ever assert this statement as absolute gospel truth, but more so begins to plant the seed in people's minds that the government might not be telling us the whole story and that there might be a malicious motive behind it.

In a story on how the United States tends to quantify the number of undocumented immigrants, Carlson uses a similar method. He begins by quoting Robert Groves, director of the Census Bureau, who apparently said, "There is no magic bullet that anyone has discovered to count [undocumented immigrants]. This is really very difficult to estimate." He goes on to slowly and carefully reveal that, in his mind anyway, there's a faulty assumption at the center of the calculation of 11 million undocumented immigrants that many politicians cite: "So many of the studies projecting that there are only 11 million illegal immigrants have in fact acknowledged that the census is not perfect, they've been honest about that. But strangely they assumed that it was pretty close to perfect. Specifically, they operated on the assumption that only about 10% of illegal immigrants weren't being captured by census takers, weren't responding to the forms. Put another way, their models assumed that 90% of the people living in this country illegally were willing to cooperate with census takers. Now why would they assume that? That seems like a ridiculous assumption. But there's a reason." If true, his reasoning does not seem outlandish here, and he does throw in some numbers, which makes his argument seem more grounded. The problem once again is his assigna-tion of a malicious motive to the operation. He slowly works up to that state-ment, "But there's a reason," upon which his more collected persona turns on a dime. Now more in the realm of suspicion and conspiracy theorizing, he suggests that this assumption rests on a left-leaning determination to make the number of undocumented immigrants in this country seem lower than it is.

Carlson is not alone in this type of mainstreaming of extremist ideas and unfounded suspicions. His colleague Laura Ingraham utilizes similar tactics to sow doubt on her popular *Fox News* show *Ingraham Angle.* At the outset, it looks like Ingraham is simply posing innocent questions. In one episode from April 2020, she shares the latest data supposedly from the Institute of Health Metrics and Evaluation (IHME), which projects the number of ventilators and ICU beds needed at COVID peaks. Somewhere in the middle of her monologue about why these new estimates are more accurate than the information we already have on the subject, she poses her central question: "Why didn't the experts know the numbers were wrong?" In the settings of these *Fox News* shows, these types of questions are never innocent. They are designed to sow doubt about the true ex-tent of the expertise of those leading the pandemic response. But just like Tucker Carlson, she works her way up to this question relatively slowly, using real sources to make her argument, before unraveling eve-rything into a hard-hitting conglomeration of conspiracy and paranoid thinking.[30]

To take a few more examples from Ingraham's show, we can look to her June 2021 treatment of vaccination, herd immunity, and natural immunity. She starts by trying to legitimize her own show by highlighting the "expert" guests she has had on since the start of the pandemic: "Over the past 16 months, *The Angle* has showcased some of the brightest minds in science and medicine, who've weighed in with meticulous precision on how best to balance health concerns (and they're very serious that were presented by this virus) against the broader economic, educational, and social needs of our citizens. Treating physicians told us about ways to effectively treat the virus early and cheaply." Make no mistake, she seems to be saying, this show has a place at the table. But after legitimizing her own work, she moves swiftly into conspiratorial thinking: "Then on herd immunity, Fauci admitted to lying about the threshold level for political reasons. He didn't want people to forgo mitigation or the vaccine." She takes a step from suggesting experts might be wrong to suggesting they might be willfully misleading the public in part to encourage greater uptake of the vaccine. She suggests that the mainstream media are hiding particular studies that, in her mind, suggest the superiority of natural to vaccinated immunity: "Look, if we had an independent and honest media, this new Cleveland study would be leading every nightly newscast. But like Fauci, they've committed to the lie that every American must be vaccinated or be made into social pariahs."[31] This suggestion that the media are purposely suppressing information in order to encourage medical innovations such as the vaccine is also conspiratorial in nature. Once again, she does not begin with these conspiracy theories, as a traditional charismatic leader might, but instead works up to them and enhances them by arguing for her mainstream legitimacy first.

Before espousing actual conspiracy theories and suspicious modes of thinking, Ingraham tries to highlight her belief that she is "open" to a wide range of ideas about any given topic. In a show from April 2020 about hydroxychloroquine, Ingraham poses a series of questions about the drug and the now-accepted scientific fact that it does not work against COVID:

Is this a mad impulse to discount any benefit from the therapy? Is it triggered by pure hatred of Trump, of Fox, of me? I don't know. Is it motivated by a secret desire to keep America hopeless or the shutdown going on through the election? I'm open to any theory at this point. If the impulse was purely scientific and health-focused, why haven't we seen the same volume of coverage and scrutiny of other, far more expensive, and also no controlled completely double-blind study of unproven treatments?[32]

Her insistence that she is "open to any theory" is an attempt to convince listeners that she is not biased. Her questions are leading, though—they suggest that there is a nefarious motive here and a concerted attempt to keep evidence about hydroxychloroquine's effectiveness away from the public by not funding any gold standard randomized trials. In the same breath, however, she puts forth some more squarely suspicious thinking about Big Pharma: "Well of course hydroxychloroquine as we've said before is cheap, it's highly scalable, it's been around for decades and decades and decades. Big Pharma does not make its money on cheap generics." She ends on the idea that liberals are in some way protecting Big Pharma's interests by insisting that hydroxychloroquine doesn't work and promoting more expensive treatments that benefit Big Pharma, in the process keeping secrets and potentially life-saving technologies from the American public. But she does not express this idea right off the bat—she works up to it by softening her audience, emphasizing her reasonableness and her lack of bias.

A similar pattern can be seen in the rhetoric of many conservative politicians. In the midst of professing a wide range of conspiracy theories, Ted Cruz is always quick to tell people that he's open to ideas from both sides of the political aisle and that he thinks it's healthy to exchange ideas. In a September 2020 appearance on the show *The View*, Cruz is quick to deploy the conspiracy theory that New York's governor at the time, Andrew Cuomo, sent COVID-positive patients to nursing homes. Yet amidst what cannot be seen as anything other than a conspiracy theory, Cruz defends himself and his extreme views by seemingly embracing everyone from all backgrounds: "Look, I recognize that the hosts of this show, y'all's politics are different from mine. And I think it's actually good we're having a conversation. Too often, left and right don't talk to each other and we just kinda yell at each other."[33] Cruz comes out looking somewhat better than the hosts of *The View*, who argue vociferously against his misinformation. We'll see that this is a common tactic of Cruz's—appearing calm and balanced while he spreads misinformation and conspiracy theories.

Early in the pandemic, Cruz took it somewhat seriously and even exhorted the American public and politicians in Washington not to use the virus as a political weapon. This attitude, particularly giving the virus its due as a serious threat, was not exactly in line with President Trump's initial downplaying of the gravity of the situation. In March 2020, in the very early days of the pandemic, Cruz self-imposed quarantine after being exposed to someone with the virus, even though the CDC, Health and Human Services (HHS), and his own doctor advised him that he didn't really meet the criteria since the exposure was extremely brief and happened nine days prior. Out of an abundance of caution, however, Cruz confined himself to his home for two weeks. When discussing the experience on *ABC News* and asked about criticism of the roll-out of COVID-19 testing, which had not gone well, he simply commented, "Don't use this as a political football for one side or the other to advance their partisan objectives."[34] On the face of it, in this interview in March 2020, Cruz comes off as a reasonable person with legitimate concerns about the virus and a plea that it not be unnecessarily politicized.

However, we know that this sort of even-keeled non-partisan calm is not his primary mode of operation. Cruz turned out to be one of the worst propagators of conspiracy theories and misinformation as the pandemic wore on, especially once Joe Biden assumed the presidency. But this is not the only time we see Cruz putting on airs. He often plays the role of the calm, even-keeled, non-partisan senator who is only trying to elicit facts and pay homage to science. In a *Fox News* interview in July 2021, only a little over a year after Cruz's self-imposed quarantine and plea that the public take the virus seriously, we see him peddling in obvious conspiracy theories, such as the idea that the feds were knowingly releasing infected migrants into the population and covering it up. He also rails against the new CDC ruling that vaccinated people should wear masks indoors, which came about largely due to the new and more infectious Delta variant against which the vaccines did not protect as well. The basis for his criticism of this new ruling, or so he says, is essentially that he believes it is not scientific:

> And at the same time, yesterday we saw the CDC issue an absurd new ruling, a ruling that people who have been vaccinated have to wear masks indoors. I gotta say, that ruling is 100% politics, it's not science, it's politics, and it shows the hypocrisy of Democrats that they want to control and restrict your freedom as Americans but at the same time they're allowing COVID-positive illegal immigrants to come into this country with no constraints at all.[35]

He views this new recommendation by the CDC as in some way "political," with his logic unfolding that he believes the Democrats are behind the

CDC and that they are also the ones who have released infected migrants into the population. How can they try to mandate that we be more restricted in efforts to combat the virus when they willingly expose us to new, covert threats?

In his February 2022 testimony before the Senate about COVID vaccine mandates, Cruz continued to harp on this idea of listening to the science, rather than pandering to politics. In response to a question about Trump touting the (nonexistent) benefits of using hydroxychloroquine to treat COVID, he responded:

> I think this is a very strange time politically where everything is viewed through a partisan and political lens. I can tell you personally I've spoken to multiple doctors who are treating large numbers of patients with COVID, multiple doctors have told me in Texas that prescribing hydroxychloroquine and zinc and azithromycin that they've seen really positive results. Now you asked me personally, I have no idea, I'm not a doctor, no one in their right mind would take my medical advice and what's strange about this is, in today's political environment, everything is viewed through a lens of Trump. Because Trump said positive things about hydroxychloroquine, suddenly a lot of the Left, a lot of the media said oh my God it's the worst thing on earth, you can't prescribe it.[36]

He continued with these themes throughout, saying things like, "My view is simple. We oughta listen to sound science, we oughta listen to medical science," and "I think people are more interested in common sense and actually trying to solve these things rather than everything being a political gladiatorial match." By focusing on these slogans about the value of science over politics, Cruz endlessly tries to legitimize himself as a reasonable, fact-based person, rather than appearing as a politician overly influenced by partisanship. But this only paves a smooth road for slices of extremist views to come out in between these statements.

Cruz most certainly does not shy away from conspiracy theories. His most oft-cited one is about the supposed release of coronavirus from a lab in Wuhan, but he also voices suspicious thoughts about Fauci and the idea that Pfizer and the government withheld vaccine efficacy data until after the November 2020 election in an elaborate plot to disadvantage Trump. He is a little less circumspect on his podcast, *The Verdict*, than he is on national media sources (other than *Fox News* for the most part). On episode 18 of that show, he has an extensive foray into his beliefs about the Wuhan Institute of Virology:

> Of all the cities on planet earth, it certainly raises some questions why the outbreak occurs where there is a government lab controlled by the government of China that's doing research and not just research into infectious diseases—it's doing research into coronaviruses that have been transmitted through bats.... So here's where the media has been super defensive—when anyone asks this question the media, like the *Washington Post* did this big hit piece saying this is a crazy conspiracy theory because they say, and I've been told by multiple scientists this, there's no evidence that this virus was constructed in a lab. Listen I have no reason to doubt that, that's what the scientists have told me and I don't know about DNA sequencing, I'm not a scientist.

Here we see something that Cruz does a lot—he espouses a more extremist theory and then he backs away from it by reminding people that he is not an authority or the most knowledgeable person on the topic. But we know that once an idea is out there, even if doubt is immediately cast upon it, it may have an influence on people's thoughts and beliefs. What Cruz engages with in these instances is more a rhetorical turn than a genuine change of heart. As he plants the seed about these types of ideas, he also returns to and repeats them, as in episode 24 of his podcast when he states: "The US government was funding the Chinese research at the Wuhan Institute of Virology.... Every one, ABC, CBS, NBC, CNN, they make millions of dollars every single year from access to China. They're terrified, they're terrified of ticking off the Chinese." This is a more forceful expression of the same idea, with more detail about the media added to explain to people why this conspiracy has not been uncovered. Slowly, he builds his case.

Cruz has spouted conspiracy theories about Fauci as well, who has been a common target of right-wing hate from the first moment he contradicted Trump. In a July 21, 2021, address to the Senate, Cruz takes aim at Fauci as part of a long complaint against the CDC's new (at the time) mask mandate for vaccinated individuals:

> I believe the CDC's decision yesterday [to mandate masks indoors for vaccinated people] was politics. It wasn't science.... The CDC months ago

rightly concluded that vaccinated people don't need to wear masks because the whole purpose of a vaccine is not to get the disease. That decision was right, the science hasn't changed. The only thing that has changed is the politics. . . . Today the credibility of the CDC is in tatters. Because leadership of the CDC has been willing to allow science to become politicized. . . . I might remind you that Anthony Fauci in those emails asked Facebook to silence anyone who said anything different than the government directive on speech, including if you suggest that the origin of the Wuhan virus was actually in Wuhan, China in a Chinese government lab. And Facebook willingly complied, censored that view.

Here we see a nice combination of Cruz's tendencies in speaking about health and scientific issues and particularly in opining on policy decisions surrounding COVID-19. In the same breath, he accuses the CDC of not being "scientific" enough, of being excessively political, while he also takes aim at Fauci, with a series of conspiracy theories that speak to his own political gain. He couches his conspiratorial thought in a veneer of scientific and supposedly apolitical calm.

Cruz also seemed to subscribe to the conspiracy theory that the Democrats made the pharmaceutical companies wait to announce positive results from their vaccine trials until after Biden won the election. In an episode of *The Verdict*, Cruz said: "What a crock. What an . . . okay that pissed me off. Pfizer literally the week after the election said hey look we cured it now . . . they couldn't have announced it the week before the election? Of course they could have. Look it's Big Pharma being totally in the tank for the Democrats, I mean it was nakedly political."[37] So he criticizes the other side for being too political, for taking action in the form of conspiracies that serve their political goals. At the same time, he claims to hold himself to a higher standard that goes beyond virtue signaling identity politics: "Y'know, it's hard to understand the politics . . . y'know listen when it comes to masks, I've never been one that's a zealot on either side, I've never really understood some of the folks who say never wear a mask no matter what . . . but I also never understood the purist who would ostentatiously wear a mask as a symbol of their nobility and purity and virtue."[38] Eschewing extremists on both sides, Cruz definitively crafts himself as a not-too-political centrist whose main responsibility supposedly lies in getting everyone else around him to stick to the facts. If you're thinking that that's not how Cruz operates as a politician in reality, you are exactly right. The point is, this kind of posturing, interspersed with heavy, very real conspiratorial tones, is basically the style lately of Republican politicians.

Turning to someone more outwardly extremist for a moment, Marjorie Taylor Greene still likes to play dumb when it comes to whether or not she espouses conspiracy thinking. Greene is educated—she went to the University of Georgia and she earned a business degree, so she is not actually as ignorant as she pretends to be at times. In 2017, she started writing for conspiracy theory and propaganda websites, engaging especially with conspiracy theories about school shootings. She is anti-Semitic and Islamophobic. She also believes in Pizzagate (a conspiracy theory that purported that a number of high-ranking U.S. officials were engaged in child trafficking in partnership with restaurants, including Comet Ping Pong Pizzeria in Washington, D.C.) and is generally a QAnon supporter. Just before Biden's inauguration, Greene sent a text to White House Chief of Staff Mark Meadows suggesting that Trump enact martial law: "In our private chat with only Members, several are saying the only way to save our Republic is for Trump to call for Marshall [sic] law. I don't know on those things. I just wanted to tell you. They stole this election. We all know. They will destroy our country next. Please tell him to declassify as much as possible so we can go after Biden and anyone else!"[39] When Greene was approached on the street by CNN's Jim Acosta about this text, she seemed to want to draw attention to her line, "I don't know on those things." Playing dumb here seemed to be her way out of the full gravity of these statements, which, if taken seriously, basically represent a threat to the peaceful transfer of power. It is interesting and telling that Greene planted this phrase in her text, in part of course because it helps exonerate her, but also because it is in keeping with the kind of half-hearted distancing from conspiracy theories that many Republicans display. As we look at more and more of these types of exchanges and interviews with Republican politicians, this form of grappling with conspiracy theories emerges as quite common and likely as a strategy to appeal to a broader, less extreme portion of the population.

We Are Not Truth Seekers

A 2021 study by van Prooijen and colleagues showed that people who endorsed conspiracy theories at time 1 of the survey used in the study (April 2020) were more likely to have been rejected by friends and other social contacts by time 2 (December 2020). Loss of social support seems to be associated with high levels of conspiracy beliefs, and it is much more likely for people espousing these beliefs to be rejected by their peers than for people with high levels of conspiracy beliefs to reject those with low levels of these beliefs. This social rejection ultimately contributes to conspiracy theory belief, as isolation is often a key factor in subscribing to these notions in the first place.[40] In fact, although it might seem like a paradox that I noted earlier that social groups reinforce conspiracy theories and now I am arguing that isolation is a key factor, it is still helpful to see these two phenomena in tandem. Take the following example: a person who recently retired or lost their job feels isolated at home all day. As a way to get some more human interaction, this person might spend time on social media sites. Gradually, as does happen on social media, they might come across conspiratorial thoughts. If they find that these ideas come with groups that offer the camaraderie they might be missing, they are more likely to join in than if they are not feeling isolated to begin with.

Van Prooijen's work suggests that casting out most people who subscribe to conspiracy theories might make things worse. While it is often difficult to deal interpersonally with someone who insists that COVID is a hoax and refuses to get a life-saving vaccination, on a societal level, we need to do a better job of accounting for and understanding the modern-day conspiracist. As I have shown throughout this chapter, conspiracy theories in the wake of COVID-19 are far more complex than they are often given credit for: they are sometimes milder on the face of things, but, more importantly, they are created and recreated through an iterative process that has pulled in more of the people on the edges, on the fences, who might not otherwise have come to believe in conspiracy theories. This is where the idea that the most powerful predictor of believing in a conspiracy theory is believing in another conspiracy theory may not be entirely accurate or applicable.

In addition, we have seen how politicians and political newscasters, mostly on the right, have preyed on people's uniquely high level of uncertainty and isolation during the pandemic by littering their rhetoric with bite-sized, less extreme, more mainstream versions of even the most "out-there" conspiracy theories. And then you have QAnon, the pinnacle of the modern conspiracy theory, with no charismatic leader to guide extreme levels of thinking and more latitude for people to adapt these outrageous beliefs and turn them into ideas that suit their own identities and self-image.

This is where I come to disagree with Uscinski and Parent and perhaps several others who have argued that conspiracy theories are not on the rise. I would argue that perhaps the "purest" forms of conspiracy theories—that there was an organized plot to kill JFK or that Princess Diana's death was staged—may not be more prevalent. What we do seem to be seeing is a wider range of people who have accepted bits and pieces of conspiracy theories into their everyday thinking. These people may distrust the COVID vaccine because of some vague sense that the pandemic is not real, but they might not openly identify with a statement that outright says that the pandemic is a global, inter-governmental plot. It is these people who may casually engage with the idea that Democrats are morally decrepit without endorsing Pizzagate. Our political moment, the rise of social media, and the extraordinary circumstances of a pandemic that unfolded in an already highly polarized nation have created this new type of "casual" conspiracy theorist. On the one hand, this is bad news: conspiracy theories have become mainstream and have infected the lifeblood of the nation. On the other hand, if these views are milder and more "casual" and perhaps somewhat even unconscious, perhaps there are greater points of intervention than we realized. As one interviewee said of his sister-in-law: "She espoused QAnon beliefs without even knowing it. If she'd known, she would've been horrified." Perhaps it is time that more people knew.

Studying the structure and nature of the modern-day, post-COVID conspiracy theory shows us that it is something quite different, something designed to go mainstream. And the circumstances of COVID, with its accompanying uncertainty, were the perfect setting for this type of conspiracy theorizing to take hold. In the next chapter, I will examine just how the government's response to COVID-19 made these circumstances even worse than they had to be and created a perfect storm for medical mistrust to erupt. In the meantime, this quote from Friedman and colleagues is apt: "We are cognitively hardwired for plausibility, not for truth or accuracy."[41(pp3–4)] Most people are not looking for the truth. They are looking for what "feels" right. If it happens to be true, that's perhaps a bonus. But human beings, as a rule, are not truth-seekers.

4

Heartbreak and Outrage

The Response to COVID-19

In January 2023, I received an email from someone who heard about my book and wanted to tell me her story. The email was full of pathos. In it, she discussed how much she loved her son and yet how heartbroken she was that he had suddenly lost faith in health and medicine and refused to get himself or his children vaccinated against COVID. Before the pandemic, she described her son as a science lover who relished in astronomy, physics, and biology. Now, he was blaming Fauci for lying about the vaccine. How did this happen? This story was not unique among the ones I heard in my interviews, and they were all equally heartbreaking. They showed me something very important—yes, that medical mistrust after COVID is a more widespread phenomenon, but also that it has taken on a different character, a kind of all-encompassing suspicion that goes beyond the health arena. In this chapter, I will elucidate what went wrong in the COVID response that has brought us to a place of such widespread and categorically different mistrust.

The inadequacy of the U.S. response to the COVID-19 pandemic does not represent a unique or entirely unexpected phenomenon. Several aspects of our failure to respond properly to the virus have to do with uniquely American traits related to our social philosophies and our healthcare system. Our failure to get the virus under control has a lot to do with widespread poor access to healthcare in this country and the concept of medical mistrust that I have been exploring throughout this book. The connection between poor access and mistrust only strengthened during the pandemic and became a key aspect of people's inability to get tested and treated and their refusal, in many cases, to get themselves and their children vaccinated. In addition to this deeply systemic issue with poor access to our healthcare system and its intimate connection with medical mistrust, there were other aspects of our response that make sense in the context of American social values, such as our reliance on the individual and our resistance to centralized authority. Both of these aspects of American social philosophy made a proper response to the pandemic infinitely more challenging. The communication failures paramount in this pandemic response are concerning on their own and, even more disturbing, represent symptoms of a failing democracy. No longer simply an issue of scientists and medical professionals being poorly trained to translate complex scientific notions into comprehensible language, the failure of political communication in this instance signals the widening gap between political powers and the populace, as well as a shattering of the foundations of public trust in political institutions that are so fundamental to democratic principles. The subsequent rise in conspiracy theories thus became a reaction to this societal crumbling and lack of trust in all of our institutions.

Before I get to how the response to the COVID pandemic in the United States might reflect the failure of many of our democratic institutions, I want to detail how exactly the response failed. On the most basic level, the Trump administration squandered time, and time of course is the most precious commodity during an infectious disease outbreak. If we are always trying to catch up to the virus, we have already lost. There are many actions that the Trump administration could and should have taken during March and April of 2020 when the pandemic was in its early days, including: instilling a culture of hand hygiene and mask-wearing; creating a supply chain and implementation infrastructure to support scaled-up utilization of diagnostics and tracing and isolation activities; devising intelligent plans to safely open schools; and investing in and testing effective public communication.[1] None of these actions was taken—instead, there was a lot of confusion about whether to wear masks, what guidelines were in place and whether or not they were required, and what responsibilities fell to the states versus the federal government. There was no early investment in the supply chain and no deep understanding of the testing process and supply needs around testing and tracing, so the early response to the pandemic, which set the stage for the outcomes of the rest of the response to the pandemic, was completely inadequate.

In conversation with infectious disease expert Céline Gounder, who also became a White House advisor on pandemic response, she added that our data systems were woefully unprepared to help us understand what was truly going on in the early days of the pandemic. In addition, she felt there were too many politicians involved in the work that public health experts should have been doing: communicating with the public. Health communications expert Heidi Tworek also suggested that the lack of a coordinated federal response was an issue from the start.

There were also some basic tenets of crisis communication that the Trump administration and his scientific advisors either did not (or did not want to) understand or heed. For example, there was no clear timetable for isolation communicated, and while it makes sense that this might have been difficult given how little we knew about the virus, its incubation period, and the period of infectivity of a positive case, even these uncertainties could have been better communicated. Encouraging people to quarantine and isolate with no clear guidelines on time limits can make people feel like their liberty is being attacked. Personal freedom is extremely important to Americans, so better communication about the time boundaries on these behaviors would have been helpful. As Tworek also noted, containment measures were communicated as restrictions rather than as tools, which raised the level of suspicion and resistance. In addition, we have never had and still do not have a good framework in this country for protection of personal data on various technology platforms, so people were understandably afraid of contact tracing apps. Americans are sensitive to personal privacy, although perhaps not as sensitive as our European counterparts. Nonetheless, contact-tracing apps were widely used in places like Germany, where there are clearer boundaries around, and public understanding of, personal privacy protection on commonly used technologies.[1]

The poor response to the pandemic started long before the pandemic itself began, with the lack of infrastructure and funding to manage large-scale public health emergencies and the communal undervaluing of public health and prevention that has been part of the hallmark American obsession with biomedical intervention. There were numerous Trump-era budget cuts to the CDC and other public health agencies that demonstrated this trend, especially in the Republican Party. In 2018, funding for CDC epidemic work was cut by 80%, and the agency scaled back its focus and research into emerging infectious diseases in several hotspots, including China. It is unsettling to think that future pandemics might arise in part from our lack of foresight in investigating other emerging infectious diseases.[2] The unsatisfactory social safety net we already have was also heavily cut under the Trump administration. There were many pre-pandemic Trump-era cuts to funding sources that protect people who are unemployed, which became problematic during the pandemic.[2] These votes of non-confidence in our primary mechanisms of pandemic and public health emergency response and in our social safety net became sites of anxiety, contention, and serious handicap once an actual pandemic took charge of our lives.

When it came to emergency and crisis communication, the Trump administration and response team did not leave anyone feeling particularly comforted. Two central tenets of good crisis communications are often at odds with each other: an unwavering commitment to transparency and stability of message. This can be difficult in light of a novel disease where information is constantly changing, but part of building trust is always being transparent about the fact that guidance has changed and why. Some people will lose trust at these junctures, but most will feel comforted by the additional explanation. As Tworek pointed out, the most important piece of communication in this type of situation is to say: the one thing we do know for sure is that we do not know everything and things will change. That was not made explicitly and regularly clear enough.

Of paramount importance during a crisis is for leaders to actively communicate shared social values.[3] Some of the traditional American social values, such as autonomy, independence, and limits to the federal government's power, might be at odds with pandemic response. Nonetheless, leaders could still communicate about these values while being transparent about situations in which these ideals may need to take a back seat. It should also go without saying that blaming and shaming, a favorite of Trump, are not useful tactics. They often lead to lower compliance. Giving people as much autonomy as possible and continually emphasizing shared goals is a much better strategy.[3] Just as leaders need to be trusted by the population, it is helpful if the reverse is also true: leaders must show that they trust the populace.[3] This might come in the form of giving people autonomy, praising them for complying to guidelines, or even saying and repeating that they trust them. Finally, another element of crisis communications 101: it should always be abundantly clear who is leading the response, and it should only be one person (or entity).[4] At the very beginning of the COVID-19 pandemic, it was unclear whether the federal government or the states were supposed to be leading the charge. Shortly thereafter, Trump put together a COVID taskforce with Mike Pence, his vice president, at the helm, but this ultimately seemed like window dressing. As we will see later in this chapter, Pence was never given the authority to act on his own, and he never spoke with the resolve of a true leader.

Our Uniquely American Failed Response

While it may be true that many countries had a less-than-optimal response to the COVID-19 pandemic, there are many ways in which our failures in the

United States are bound up in some of the structural and political features of our country's inner workings. Robert Schneider, author of *An Unmitigated Disaster: America's Response to COVID-19*, has argued that our response to the pandemic failed in part due to the social ideal and, in many ways, holy grail of American culture: individualism.[5] Even before the mayhem of the past few years and the pandemic response, Americans' general level of distrust of government institutions has always been high. Part of the reason for that is that there has always been a strong preference for individual over government action. Well before COVID, Alexis de Tocqueville opined that there were three major features of American democracy: tyranny of the majority, individualism, and despotism.[5(p52)] Both individualism and tyranny of the majority, seemingly disparate concepts though actually quite similar in their disregard for centralized government authority, are absolute disasters during a pandemic. A crisis such as a pandemic requires coordination and firm control from a centralized authority. It is not a time when the opinions of the majority should be primarily honored, but rather a time when a small band of experts must lead the response. In this way, we have seen the tyranny of the majority gain even more ground in recent years, with the distaste for expertise and highly concentrated centers of power in Washington.

De Tocqueville also commented that Americans feel no debt to the past and no sense of obligation to the future.[5(p52)] In this account, Americans have always had an inclination toward "presentism," rather than a sense of duty to bring past ideals and values into play, or a concern for a future that goes beyond the next few months or years. Indeed, short-sightedness has been a feature of many of our responses to recent policy challenges, our treatment of the environment and our response to climate change being chief examples among them.

In characterizing America's response to the pandemic, Schneider also calls upon a seminal work by Richard Hofstadter, *Anti-Intellectualism in American Life*.[5(p52)] In this tome, Hofstadter argues that anti-intellectualism is a key part of American life and a key part of American culture. For Hofstadter, this anti-intellectualism was intimately tied with utilitarianism, a sense that rational thought and behavior are valued insofar as they contribute to utility and minimization of pain, but that knowledge in and of itself is not of too much value. The idea is that knowledge is only valuable inasmuch as it enhances personal well-being and self-interest.[5(p52)]

So cultural and social values relating to individualism and self-interest certainly hindered the pandemic response. There were also structural features of American governance that hindered a proper pandemic response.

As most people know, the United States operates in a federalist system in which power is mostly decentralized and allocated to individual states. There is not necessarily anything inherently wrong with this approach. As Schneider points out, the cascading of power from the president all the way to the local level, which is how our public health system operates, is a sensible and useful structure in a crisis. Contact tracing is most effective when it is implemented by a trusted local authority rather than the nameless, shapeless "big government." In addition, while trust in centralized government authority has eroded in recent years, trust in local authorities such as local public health officials was still quite high at the start of the pandemic.[5(p52)] Assurance of privacy as part of a strategy like contact tracing is easier when this activity is conducted at the local level, in part because small pockets of data are less valuable to hackers than large government databases.

But our piecemeal response ended up being nothing short of a disaster. There was a massive failure of governance, in which states were never clear where to look for guidance on what they actually had the authority to do.[5(p52)] Our federalist system often gave states free reign to craft their own responses to COVID, but most of the time they did not have the economic resources to carry their plans to fruition.[5(p61)] As a result, they almost never had the full set of supplies they needed and crippling shortages were common. In an ideal world, federalist systems are marked by tiering of responsibilities and authorities, including federal responsibility to maintain harmony among states, primacy of the legislative branch, federal responsibility for equal protection of the laws, and devolution of power.[1] Public health is always the domain of the state, not the federal government, except in cases of interstate commerce, national security, or regulation of external borders. In all these cases, the federal government is permitted to take some action and oversee the situation with more authority. Interstate commerce is often involved in public health matters, so there needs to be a careful coordination between state, local, and federal authorities.[1(p66)] As a result, public health response is quite complex and multilayered.

In the case of COVID-19, interstate commerce was certainly relevant, and the federal government needed to play some part in the response, even while allowing states freedom to act on their own. In the case of an infectious disease that obviously crosses state borders easily, the federal government in many cases had jurisdiction to act on the states' behalf. One of the missteps early in the pandemic was a failure of the federal government to control resource allocation to states. Engendering a kind of free-market philosophy that is not appropriate during a national emergency, the federal government sat back and mostly allowed states to "fend for themselves" when it came to securing crucial supplies such as personal protective equipment (PPE) and ventilators. States began to bid against each other, entering an interstate trade war. This competition for resources quickly became a threat to the peaceful functioning of the federalist system. In this case, the federal government should have supplied resources to states directly and also should have provided surge capacity to states.[1] They also should have defined minimally acceptable standards for COVID testing and social distancing protocols that states had to follow. The federal government is entrusted with the authority to ensure that one state's actions do not threaten the well-being of another state, which is partially why the federal government must get involved in cases of interstate commerce.[1(p81)]

In the media, both at the time and later upon reflection, there was a lot of talk about how the fragmented nature of the federalist system doomed the pandemic response from the start. There have been many statements about how our healthcare and public health systems are fundamentally ill-equipped to manage a health crisis of national and international concern, mostly because of the federalist system.[6-10] I think many of these statements require some degree of qualification. It is true that in this case, there was a fragmented response with a lack of desperately needed federal oversight. Yet, we cannot assume based on the failure of our response to COVID that the federalist system is necessarily ill-equipped to handle a national emergency. The federalist system is actually quite an elegant structure that allows for a neutralizing, equalizing force (the federal government) to oversee the mostly independent actions and plans of a state government. The problem is that it may be too easy to take advantage of the federalist structure, whether the reason might be to allow the federal government to step away from the problem or to allow capitalist forces to function unencumbered.

Trump himself constantly changed positions on who had the authority to enact public health measures in individual states. In one of his early daily briefings on COVID on April 13, 2020, Trump declared: "The President of the United States has the authority to do what the President has the authority to do, which is very powerful. The President of the United States calls the shots. If we weren't here for the states, you would've had a problem in this country like you've never seen before, we were here to back them up and we've more than backed them up, we did a job that nobody ever thought was possible."[11] At the same briefing, he also argued: "When someone's the

President of the United States, their authority is total, and that's the way it's gotta be . . . the authority of the President of the United States having to do with the subject we're talking about is total."[11] Yet just three days earlier, at another briefing on April 10, 2020, the president conceded his authority to the state: "I like to allow governors to make decisions without overruling them because from a Constitutional standpoint that's the way it should be done. If I disagreed, I would overrule a governor, and I have that right to do it, but I'd rather have them—you could call it federalist, you could call it the Constitution, but I call it the Constitution—I would rather have them make their decision."[12] Calling upon our county's federalist structure and invoking the Constitution, here Trump seems to argue that any kind of authority he has is diluted by the states' power of self-governance. In reality, he tended to declare total control whenever he wanted to take credit for a success, and leave things up to the state whenever he wanted to evade a question. If someone asked about shortages of supplies in certain states or why certain states were not following social distancing guidelines, he would generally invoke federalism and the Constitution. There were constant questions about why states were bidding against each other for ventilators if, as Trump often insisted, there were enough to go around from those supplied by the federal government. In response to one such question at an April 2, 2020, briefing, Trump said:

> They have to work that out. What they should do, what they should've been doing is long before this pandemic arrived, they should've been on the open market just buying, there was no competition, you coulda made a great price. The states have to stock up. It's like one of those things—they waited, they didn't want to spend the money because they thought this would never happen, and their shelves in some cases were bare. . . . So the best thing they can do is when times become normalized and they will be hopefully soon . . . they oughtta stock up for the next time.[13]

It is easy and natural to throw up one's hands in frustration at such obvious evasion of responsibility. What is notable here, however, is not necessarily that Trump hides behind federalism to shirk responsibility, but rather that he speaks in a manner that is consistent with a quintessentially American response to the situation. His overreliance on capitalism, self-regulation, and a form of unencumbered "healthy" competition, is actually nothing new. It is part of the very fabric of the American enterprise and demonstrates the many ways in which the response to this pandemic was, in fact, a very American affair.

Even more respected experts in infectious disease who became some of the president's spokespeople on the scientific aspects of the virus had a similar reaction when asked about individual states' practices. In answer to questions about the situation in Florida, both Anthony Fauci and Deborah Birx demurred. During a briefing on April 10, 2020, Fauci said:

> From pure public health issues is that if you have a situation in which you don't have real great control over an outbreak and you allow children to gather together, they likely will get infected, and if they get infected, the likelihood is that they will bring the infection home, so that is a risk. I don't know the situation at all in any detail and I'm not specifically speaking about Florida, I'm just speaking generically about what happens when you have infections in the community and you have congregation of people, such as in classrooms, that that's a risk.[12]

Fauci recognizes the fact that allowing children to gather, such as at school or daycare, is a risk in any infectious disease outbreak, but how little he knows about the situation in Florida is as if someone had asked him about a country outside the United States. "I don't know the situation at all in any detail," he says, in case there is any doubt about his level of knowledge about COVID policies and outcomes in Florida.

In response to a reporter's question about myriad crowded beaches in Florida, with spring breakers and vacationers letting caution fly to the wind during an international emergency, Birx provided a similar response to Fauci's: "Well as I described, we go metro by metro, county by county, and so I'd have to link that with a specific county and look at their case rates . . . if the county health directors believe that that's appropriate for their county, then I'm not going to second-judge an individual's approach to this."[14] While part of her answer might have to do with not having the data available to her immediately at that moment, her rather political response to the question is a little jarring. In this moment, Birx sounds a little bit like Trump, not taking responsibility for whatever irresponsible behaviors might be happening in Florida and declaring that it is not her place to "second-judge" local health officials. But why do she and Fauci cling to local and state autonomy and to professed ignorance in the face of questions about the uneven response to the pandemic? Some of it might be to appear in line with Trump's approach, which, as I've already noted, was selectively federalist. More likely, especially in Fauci's case, we are seeing at play here a major failure of our public health system to operate with full functionality. The elegant structure of cascading responsibility central to our public health system is meant to delegate important tasks such as local surveillance, contact tracing, and mass administration of vaccines to the local level, where logistical handling of these matters does make more sense. It is not, however, meant to give the federal government and federal public health agencies the means to ignore irresponsible public health policies and behaviors and inconsistent enforcement of needed measures at the state and local levels. Trump was somewhat right when he said the office of the president has a certain amount of authority (perhaps not "total" authority, however, as he put it). The fragmented nature of our public health system does not mean that federal authorities cannot intervene when states and localities are not behaving in ways that promote the greater health and well-being of the nation. In this way, we saw a central tenet of American democracy abused during the U.S. response to COVID-19. In times of crisis, it is not surprising that the full function of our democracy might undergo some pressure testing. In this case, we failed the test.

Poor Access, Poor Trust

It is a core contention of democracy everywhere that the state is responsible for citizens' well-being and even their flourishing, which extends beyond mere well-being and allows people to thrive on opportunities for autonomy and self-governance.[1(p9)] There is therefore a tight connection between the functioning of public health systems and the functioning of democracy more broadly in any modern society. A society whose hospitals function poorly, for example, will experience a drop in the perceived legitimacy of political institutions as well.[1(p3)] In a democratic society, we have both positive and negative liberties. We tend to think and hear mostly about our negative liberties, including freedom of speech, freedom of the press, and freedom of religion, which all have to do with ensuring that certain rights are not taken away from us. But positive liberties are just as significant, even if they are not as widely discussed. Important ones include the ability to vote and take part in our democracy, and the ability to flourish, which depends upon a positive health state and a good economy that allows us to practice all of our negative and positive liberties.[1(p11)] COVID represented a challenge to democracy all over the world in part because the legitimacy of democracies is derived from the health and well-being of its populace, and this was brought seriously into question with this novel virus that quickly got out of control.[1(p9)]

In the 21st century, it has also emerged that societies must secure social equality and non-discrimination in addition to securing material well-being and honoring positive and negative liberties.[1(p12)] In the United States, health inequities were fully on display during the COVID crisis. If it was an option to ignore them before, it was no longer possible once COVID became widespread. Racial and ethnic minorities consistently experienced worse outcomes as a result of COVID infection.[15,16] Prior and even simultaneous efforts to undermine the Affordable Care Act (ACA) and to fight Medicaid expansion left many Americans, including some of the most vulnerable Americans, without access to healthcare during an infectious disease crisis of global proportions.[2] During a crisis, constitutional democracy survives by helping its inhabitants find a common purpose.[1(p29)] It is all too painfully obvious that finding a common purpose is difficult, to say the least, in 21st-century America. Political divisions are rife, but even putting that aside momentarily, there are also serious ruptures in our society due to inequities in access to social rights such as healthcare. The complete lack of access to healthcare in some communities has led to lower trust in pandemic guidelines and response. This has engendered a difficult set of circumstances in which even when people do get access to needed healthcare, they feel suspicious. Even under Biden, when the response to the pandemic arguably improved, only 52% of Americans report trusting public health institutions such as the CDC.[17]

Urging people to seek services they do not have access to can fuel distrust. When you tell someone to do something they cannot do as a result of structural factors beyond their control, they tend to trust you less and feel that you are blaming or shaming them, which is also a factor in feelings of trust.[18] This was a hallmark of pandemic communications, especially after funding for programs such as state-sponsored PCR testing ran out and was never renewed. Mass calls for people to get vaccinated were often met with anger and suspicion as people noted they had neither the means of transportation nor the time off work to actually obtain a vaccine. There are also certain features of the healthcare system that make it impossible to fathom a positive, coordinated response to a threat such as a pandemic. Healthcare systems like the one we have in the United States are designed to deal mostly with acute, discrete disasters, such as mass shootings and large traffic incidents. We are not well-equipped to deal with ongoing disasters that last for months or years. This is a place where there may have been a kernel of truth in Trump's complaints about the "stockpile" he inherited, although the degree to which he blamed the Obama administration for this was unfounded. Not surprisingly, because of the focus on discrete disasters, there was not enough substance to our public health response. Early responses to the pandemic focused almost entirely on the hospitalized population and failed to deal adequately with community spread.[8] This pattern is typical of the U.S. healthcare system in general, in which a premium is placed on downstream medical intervention as opposed to upstream public health methods of prevention. Putting all of these factors together, the inequities and poor access to care, leading to distrust in the healthcare and public health systems, our political divisions that prevented the country from coming together in order to protect our constitutional democracy, and the narrow focus on medical rather than public health–oriented interventions already extant in our healthcare system, it becomes obvious why our response has been so inadequate.

In his daily briefings on the pandemic in the early days, then-President Trump liked to harp on what he perceived as a dwindling stockpile that he supposedly inherited from his predecessor. At a briefing on April 13, 2020, he said: "We inherited a stockpile where the cupboards were bare. There was nothing. . . . Just like we didn't have ammunition, we didn't have medical supplies, we didn't have ventilators, we didn't have a lot of things that should've been had." Later, during the same briefing, he repeated himself: "We rebuilt a whole industry, because we inherited nothing. What we inherited from the previous administration was totally broken . . . not only were the cupboards bare, as I say, but we inherited broken testing, now we have great testing."[11] While his obsession with the previous administration seems mostly delusional, his criticism of the lack of preparation for the pandemic bears some truth. It is the case that as a country we were unprepared for a pandemic of these proportions, but it is worth pausing over the impact of the president constantly harping on this fact. Not only is it not helpful, since the issue at the center of a crisis is always going to be what should we do right now, not what should we have done four years ago, his commentary probably had the effect of drawing people's attention to the problem of access in this country. For one thing, his partisan comments are of course the absolute worst tactics during a time when the country needed to unite. Beyond this, however, there is a sense that his focus on access and supply issues may have reduced people's trust in both the healthcare and the political systems.

Americans are not stupid (for the most part). Looking, for example, at the comments section on some of Trump's early briefings, we can easily detect the total failure of people's faith in our healthcare system. As one commenter noted in the comments in response to an April 2, 2020, briefing: "Private healthcare, of which Reagan was so proud, is falling apart and on its face. It's not meant to cope with a pandemic. Fortunately, national healthcare systems ARE. Which is why the US is on its knees . . ."[13] The idea that private healthcare in this country is in no shape to "cope with a pandemic" is accurate, and in fact the piecemeal nature of our healthcare system did not help matters. Commenting on an April 17, 2020, briefing, another American citizen draws on the image of American healthcare in other countries: "YOU can see reality NOW. The world was mocking americans [sic] for decades. School system? Politics for rich? A joke as medical system? And you thought USA is the best, why?"[19] In this case, the commenter has drawn parallels with other American systems and societal ideals that are also ailing, including the school system and income inequality.

When Trump did get questions about the average American's access to healthcare during a health crisis, he faltered. At a March 26, 2020, briefing, a reporter asked him about what the administration was doing about people who had recently become uninsured due to massive job loss. His response was less than satisfactory:

> So, I mean, the things I just read to you are being considered and other things are being considered uh people are going to be getting big checks and it's not their fault, what happened to them is not their fault, so we're doing—we're doing a lot of different things on health insurance, we have meetings on it today, we're taking care of our people—this is not their fault, what happened and we're taking care. We're starting off by sending them very big checks, I think for a family of 4 it's about $3,000 and uh we're taking care of our people, we're taking care of our workers. This was not, y'know as I say, this was not a financial crisis, this was a health crisis, a medical crisis, we're gonna take care of our people.[20]

The repetitive turns of phrase in this response would not leave most Americans feeling as though their access to healthcare was secure. There is no assurance of a clear plan to manage the health of the millions of Americans who lack health insurance in the middle of an infectious disease crisis. Instead, he insists repeatedly that "we're gonna take care of our people," but how this is going to happen is still shrouded in mystery. In addition, there is an interesting theme running through Trump's remarks having to do with the placing of blame. As he mentions repeatedly, the people he is "gonna take care of" are in a situation that is "not their fault." This notion of blame and "deserving" is actually central to our healthcare system's operation in general. People "deserve" certain kinds of healthcare based on how good their employment is. Members of the population who have a higher-level employer and generally higher income enjoy generous health benefits. Wage workers and those with lower-income levels of employment that require less education often experience serious healthcare coverage gaps, if they are offered coverage at all. The connection between health insurance and employment in our country creates a tiered, hierarchical system in which the level of coverage you receive is directly tied to markers of status such as education and income. The idea that someone "deserves" or does not deserve health coverage is foreign in many countries around the world, but Trump's insistence that he will help people in this situation because they do not "deserve" what happened to them is not a foreign concept in the United States. As usual, Trump's bald and blunt style is sometimes shocking, but he is drawing on a notion that is central to the operation of American healthcare.

In this scenario, the link between access and mistrust becomes quite clear. When people have poor access to healthcare, their trust in the system begins to erode, not only because at face value it is difficult to trust a system that repeatedly shuts you out and provides you with nothing, but also because there is a psychological compensatory process that leads people to reject things they cannot have. The thought process goes something like: "Well if I can't have it, I may as well think that it is useless and corrupt and doesn't work." At the same time, often coming from a place of real desperation, people will turn to complementary and alternative medicine for the hope of a cure. Access issues did not go anywhere during the pandemic, especially toward the beginning of the crisis, and it should come as no surprise that even though there were efforts to provide free testing and ultimately free vaccines as well as financial assistance throughout the duration of the worst days of the pandemic, many Americans were still left in impossible situations. Sick and repeatedly turned away from the care and treatment they needed, their mistrust of our public health and healthcare systems deepened.

Political Communication and the Failure of Democracy

Early in the pandemic, a Health and Human Services (HHS) spokesperson accused the CDC of running a "left-wing resistance" devoted to undermining Trump.[21] Also early in the pandemic, the Trump administration barred the CDC from making the recommendation that senior citizens not travel.[21] The White House pressured the CDC regarding guidelines around reopening schools, businesses, and other venues where people gather and ultimately removed references to social distancing among younger members of the population and widespread testing and tracing.[21] In August 2020, the CDC removed guidelines about testing among asymptomatic individuals due to more pressure from Washington.[21] The Trump administration also created new protocols that required the CDC's guidelines be cleared by the Office of Management and Budget, which slowed down the release of important guidance to the general population.[21] Trump went so far as to publish his own unofficial stream of data about COVID, which was not based on any kind of real science.[21] In a frenzy of insistence on the effectiveness of a drug called hydroxychloroquine, which was quickly proven ineffective against COVID-19, Trump ordered the drug's release from a national stockpile, even though this should have been a state matter.[21] At one point, White House chief of staff Mark Meadows told the FDA commissioner Stephen Hahn that he would have to retire if the vaccine were not ready by December 11, 2020.[21] Trump repeatedly attacked and undermined inspectors general, who were charged with rolling out a response to COVID. He lashed out and replaced several of them (or tried to), including individuals who were responsible for the public health response to COVID.[21]

All of these actions represent a serious breach of power and a serious threat to our constitutional democracy. Trump, acting like a dictator, repeatedly blocked citizens' access to high-quality data and guidance that, if left intact, could most likely have saved more lives. What all these actions add up to is a translation of the COVID crisis from the public health to the political sphere. It was not the case in other, similar democratic countries, including countries in Western Europe, that political leaders ignored science and experts so much. In other comparable countries, COVID was not a hotly contested political issue.[5]

This move from public health to political sphere and the absolute control Trump tried to maintain over the narrative of the COVID crisis are symptoms of a failing democracy. The communication culture in any given society, especially as it exists at the highest levels of power, says a great deal about the health of that society's democratic institutions. In the case of the United States, both the inability to communicate effectively during a crisis and the near-totalitarian control over the flow and content of information represent a serious threat to our free society.

A new trend in communication identified in the early 21st century is still relevant today and has great relevance to the communication failures we witnessed during the pandemic. An increasing trend of anti-elitism and populism has obscured traditional party politics. A more fragmented, less homogenous audience, more dependent on social media and less dependent on traditional media, has arisen. There is also a strong social media (and somewhat of a traditional media) trend of focusing on and emphasizing identity politics over party politics.[22(p5)] This focus on identity has made political communication much more fraught than it has been in the past and has caused people to cling to certain ideologies even if they are not strongly identified with one dominant political party or the other. Some specific factors that have led to our current breakdown in political communication:

1. **Development of large, complex policy areas:** Most politicians cannot possibly understand all that is involved with modern health, economic, environmental, and technology policy. It is far too complex. As a result, most politicians do not fully understand the contents of what they are communicating, which most would agree is not a good start.

2. **Breakdown of trust in politicians and political institutions:** There will be more on this topic and how it compares to the breakdown in trust in healthcare institutions in the next chapter, but most Americans can see that there is an air of anti-elitism, anti-bureaucracy, and anti-establishment sentiment coursing through the veins of American society at the moment. The reasons for these phenomena are complex but include an increasingly crisis-driven policy environment, as we deal with multiple urgent situations including economic disasters, climate change, and epidemics; an increase in partisan politics, which has often led to a lack of progress in Washington; severe income inequality that has left many Americans feeling as though their country has abandoned or betrayed them; and a coordinated anti-elitist, anti-government, populist movement that has gained ground in establishment politics.

3. **The rise of ideologically fragmented parties**: In addition to there being growing polarization between the two main political parties, there is now also increased division within each party. This "infighting" has led to unclear and inconsistent communication, as parties often cannot decide on a unified message and policy route.

4. **Rapidly growing but unstable new parties, interest groups, and social movements**: In large part due to social media and other novel, disruptive forms of communicating and organizing, it is easier for new parties to form and gain followers. At the same time, it is easier for these parties to quickly fall apart, as they usually do not have the funding and establishment backup to hold water in Washington. Nonetheless, their formation and disbandment are disruptive to politics as usual and to political communication, as people form new opinions and hear new information (and misinformation) that may not gel with official communication and positions on various policy topics. These can lead to confusion, at best, and disbelief, distrust, and the growth of conspiracy theories, at worst.

5. **New levels of difficulty ascertaining the truth**: It is not an exaggeration anymore to say that we live in a "post-truth" world. Much of the incorrect information people confront, most of it online, originates from some form of bad actor, whether a foreign government, a local government, or a group of individuals, that deliberately spreads falsehoods. Once these falsehoods embed themselves in the flow of information on social media or even in traditional media, they are picked up and spread further, often unintentionally as misinformation. During the pandemic, the World Health Organization declared an "infodemic" in response to the poor information environment and the volume of falsehoods circulating about COVID-19. This kind of uncertainty about what is true and who can be trusted is not new, but its pervasiveness is unprecedented. This results in a situation in which the veracity of even official political communications is immediately questioned. High-quality information is often discarded as "fake news" or deliberate falsehood by those who are politically motivated.[22(pp7–8)]

All of these elements have resulted in a diversified information environment with information of varying levels of truth and rigor, in which people suddenly have the option to "choose their own adventure." If they do not like the way official government information sounds, and people often do not, they can choose not only to ignore it but to replace it with another version of reality they can easily find online.

It should not be surprising that, given the pandemic emergency and failed communications around it, many people became newly radicalized or lost trust in the healthcare system and the government. In January 2023, I spoke to one man who was still reeling from what happened. Prior to the pandemic, he had been a scientifically trained expert on vaccines, working mostly in veterinary contexts. By the time I spoke to him, he had lost his job due to his refusal to be vaccinated against COVID. He became immediately suspicious of the "warp speed" venture given his knowledge of how long it takes to develop a vaccine. Over time, he distrusted that the data coming from the government were accurate and eventually came to believe that the vaccine was a ploy for worldwide governmental control of the global population. A lot of what fueled his beliefs was what he viewed as inconsistent or misleading messaging from the CDC and other government officials. Another person told me that his father, who eventually came to believe one-world government conspiracy theories in relation to COVID-19, was always distrustful of the government but had a particularly bad reaction to the way the CDC seemed to backtrack during the pandemic. Another woman told me a close friend of hers became obsessed with conspiracy theories about the pandemic, and while before the pandemic she did have those tendencies and one could have a calm conversation with her about it, during the pandemic she would become incensed and defensive about these topics. Yet another person told me her mother's fear of vaccines increased during the pandemic and broadened her discomfort with seeking medical care. Some people would say that they trusted healthcare until they encountered Fauci.

It certainly does not help matters that local media have been decimated over the past several decades. It is now more common to live in a "media desert," in which local news simply does not exist. At the same time, local news stations have been usurped in astonishing numbers by large corporations with no background in the provision and broadcasting of quality information. Local newspapers have closed at an alarming rate, and it can be difficult for people in smaller geographic locations to have access not only to local news, but even to national news. What reaches them about national news can often be distorted through channels such as social media. At the same time, there has been a lot of consolidation of news sources, with five companies now owning one-third of the 1,400 local TV stations, and one in three local news stations not producing the content they air.[23(p221)] Most of this is a consequence of overall economic instability that has hit the news industry particularly hard.[23(p221)] Local news organizations have been taken over by large corporations with a profit motive, so a serious tension has arisen between news as a public good and news as a product.[23(p224)] To make things even worse, many of these corporations have not only a profit motive but also a political motive. Investigative reporting by all but a few high-profile newspapers, such as the *New York Times*, has basically disappeared. They have been replaced by an increased emphasis on soundbites and profiling political personalities. An important component of the free press, the ability to speak truth to power, has in many cases disappeared, as large corporations basically dictate what local media stations can and should discuss. As a result, many Americans are fed a steady diet of propaganda, instead of carefully curated and investigatively procured facts.[23(p37)] Some have argued that understanding local issues and talking to others about what to do about them is central to democracy, so the lack of exposure to local issues is hurting democracy.[23(p279)]

In general, communities need access to eight types of information: emergencies and risks; health and welfare, both local and group-specific where possible; education, including the quality of local schools; economic opportunities, including jobs, training, and small business assistance; transportation, including alternatives, costs, and schedules; the environment, including information about air and water quality, environmental threats to health, and access to restoration and recreation; civic information, including opportunities to associate with others; and political information, including information about candidates at all relevant levels of governance and public policy initiatives affecting communities and neighborhoods.[23(p35)] If we look at this list, we can discern that health information is a major component of the kind of information communities need in order to be well-informed and included appropriately in the democratic process. Emergencies and risks, health and welfare information, environmental information, educational information, and economic information can all be said to fall under the umbrella of public health, as many of these areas are social determinants of health. So the well-being of communities relies in many ways on health information. When the quality of health information is violated or manipulated, the well-being of communities is threatened on many fronts. Ultimately, the ability of a community to actualize and participate in the democratic process depends on how health messaging is delivered. And yet, uniform standards for alerting the public to imminent dangers to their health and well-being do not exist in this country.[23(p36)] At the same time, there is widespread agreement that access to high-quality information is an important predictor of social and economic outcomes.[23(p44)]

Lessons from the United Kingdom can provide some insight into what has happened to the American media in recent years. We have experienced what some have called a "mediatization of politics," in which media sources are institutionalized to the point where they actually construct reality.[24(p155)] *Fox News* provides a good example of this process—it has become more of an institution than a media source and has created the viewpoints of many Americans. As a result, government actors begin communicating differently, with a focus on spinning everything politically to gain support in the form of soundbites proliferated by the media.[24(p10)] But "political spin" can reduce trust, and of course an erosion of trust has the capacity to threaten the foundations of democracy. As political actors look to the media as a source of political gain, the boundary between political communication and simple provision of information becomes blurred.[24(p159)]

In the United Kingdom in recent years, political imperatives to manage how the media report on politics have created a centralized political communication agenda in which impartiality is increasingly difficult. Taken together with the outward fighting against career civil servants that many politicians have engaged in, we have the perfect recipe for a communication environment in which trust is low, sensationalism is high, and "truth" is increasingly difficult to discern. These factors are not unique to the United Kingdom—during the Trump administration and especially during the COVID pandemic, we saw increasing, inappropriate executive control of government employees and civil servants. For these employees, the ability to speak out and access the public became increasingly challenging. When the government cannot be trusted to communicate pertinent, important information during a crisis, when citizens have reason to believe that the government is lying or fabricating data, when opposition is explicitly silenced, and when the structure of the media does not allow for proper recourse on these abuses, we most certainly have a democracy that is in decline.

It is also helpful to understand what has been happening to our democracy in recent years, as this forms the backdrop to the breakdown in political communication we saw during the pandemic. There are two trends that many political scientists believe have contributed to the slow erosion of democratic societies: globalization and neoliberalism. Because of globalization, some capitalist institutions have grown larger than individual economies, with consequences such as climate change, international migration, and food, energy, and other resource shortages occurring outside the control of democratic institutions. This kind of lack of control over enormous changes within a society can cause a government to lose its national sovereignty and leave inhabitants feeling they are no longer citizens of a unified entity. Populism is often a reaction to globalization, with its focus on the here and now and the local country and economy over global citizenship, as evidenced by phrases such as "America first" and phenomena such as Brexit.[22(p46)]

Within the United States, party politics have also changed a great deal in recent years. There has been somewhat of a reorganization of society, with a smaller working class, less union membership, and more fragmentation across the spectrum. As discussed earlier, the sense of "local community" has mostly eroded, in part due to the closure of so many local news outlets. Politicians have shifted their attention to a more "general," national audience rather than connecting with local communities, and regional ties to particular political parties have diminished dramatically.[22(p58)] There has been a kind of "mediatization" of politics in which politicians, desperate to get national media attention, speak more in sound bites, there is much less coverage of full speeches, and less attention to the complexities of policy issues.[22(pp97–98)] In order to survive in the current political atmosphere, politicians must come up with catchy ideas, rather than necessarily engage in the full extent of policy matters. Fringe parties, with the capacity to form and disband quickly and with ease, are also more common than they have been in the past.[22(p71)]

The decline of the sense of local community, in some part due to the death of so many local news sources, and the reduction of regional ties to politics are both disastrous trends for the health of our democracy. A democracy is often in crisis when community and civic engagement drastically decline. In representative democracies, this often takes the form of decreased voting, decreased political party membership, and decreased trust in institutions, both political and otherwise.[22(p110)] The trust issue is especially germane in the United States, and trust in the healthcare system often goes hand in hand with trust (or lack of it) in a wide array of political institutions. During the COVID-19 pandemic, trust declined not only in the arena of healthcare, but also in political and government institutions as well. The failure of communication during a crisis, as witnessed especially during the early days of the COVID-19 pandemic, is really a symptom of an ailing democracy and not simply a matter of training public health professionals to communicate better. Laying all the onus on health and public health professionals misses the point and gives these professionals an impossible task of fixing a problem that is rooted much deeper than they could ever reach.

To build public confidence, government communications need to do the following: practice leadership in the national interest, rather than in personal or party interests; deliver accurate and timely information that is accessible to all; accept and respond to public scrutiny; be aware of and recognize a range of populations; show commitment to the needs of the most vulnerable; and establish a clear evidence base for statements and actions.[24(pp247–248)] It is easy to see that all of these principles were violated during the COVID-19 response under former president Trump. But this is not just a matter of Republicans versus Democrats. Many of these features of communication are still not at play under Trump's successor Joe Biden, especially when it comes to our COVID response and communications, and have become bedrocks of U.S. political communication rather than an anomaly.

During a crisis, governments are usually judged across several dimensions: capability, competence, compassion, correctness, credibility, and anticipation.[25(p11)] Capability generally refers to the fact that appropriate resources are available; competence refers to the efficient application of needed resources; compassion refers to whether communication demonstrates concern for and understanding of victims and their families; correctness refers to perceptions of honesty in communication, fairness in allocation of resources, and transparency in assistance; credibility refers to consistent and reliable provision of information; and anticipation asks whether the crisis was avoidable or if better procedures could have been in place to deal with it. Anticipation during a crisis such as the COVID-19 pandemic is also about the art of figuring out what might happen next within that same crisis (as opposed to future crises) and responding appropriately and efficiently.

It is clear that the Trump administration faltered on nearly all of these elements and that the early response to the pandemic could not have inspired much confidence in anyone. We did not have the appropriate resources available, we did not deploy them efficiently, not much compassion was shown to the victims of this terrible virus, and there was never a sense that anyone was thinking about what might come next and responding to it before it became a crisis. Most importantly for the purposes of understanding trust in public health systems and government, communication was not honest, and there was little or no attention paid to issues of equity and access. Under the Biden administration, it is still mostly the case that not enough attention is paid to issues of equity and access. Communication that is not transparent and ignores these issues is particularly prone to spiking feelings of distrust in the population. Access and trust are intimate bedfellows. When access is violated, trust deteriorates. The lack of communication about access issues and the surrounding actual lack of access that many Americans experienced and continue to experience at various points along the COVID-19 prevention, testing, and treatment pathway have created a crisis of trust and a breeding ground for conspiracy theories. All of this has occurred against a backdrop of a failing democracy, of which serious communication missteps are an ominous symptom.

Case Study: COVID-19 Press Briefings

Some of the early (and often serious) missteps in communication during the pandemic were features of the virus and our evolving knowledge of them. But some of them were secondary to Trump's self-serving, populist regime, itself a byproduct of the current moment in the history of our democracy. Some of the communication missteps have not improved much during the Biden administration. For example, in the early days, especially in the spring of 2020, there was far too much top-down communication and not enough of an attempt to reach community-based organizations and to train them in disseminating sound, evidence-based messages to community members.[26] I would argue that there is still not nearly enough of this going on, especially when it comes to historically marginalized populations, many of which might be feeling hesitant about getting vaccinated. Communication during a crisis should always be bidirectional, and governments should solicit feedback from communities on how their communications are landing.[26] It is not surprising that the Trump administration did not engage in this, given how averse Trump is to feedback, but it is also not clear that the Biden administration was engaging in this kind of feedback process either.

Part of the problem with communication during the pandemic that many people have noted is that this was a novel virus about which new data were constantly becoming available. Avoiding uncertainty and complications in communication is always a mistake—it is best to opt for transparency. In addition, and this is one that scientific and public health communicators struggle with, it is important to communicate that not all decisions are purely scientific, but that there are economic, educational, and social issues at play as well.[27] In conversation with Céline Gounder, she noted that there often was not enough demarcation in what were purely health and medical issues and decisions, and what were economic, social, or other types of issues and decisions. Good public health communication requires a concept that is at the center of this book: trust. Trust in a democracy is built on transparency and high levels of civic engagement, which is often a form of empowerment. Both of these are at all-time lows now, and were especially low during the pandemic, resulting in deep distrust of almost everything officials have said about it. In one Pew study, 57% of people said that changes in officials' recommendations about how to contain the virus made them wonder if the officials were holding back information, and only 43% said changes in officials' recommendations made them feel like they were staying on top of new information.[28] The notion that good governmental communication is built on institutional trust is in stark contrast to a deficit model, in which the government's primary objective is simply to educate the public about something they do not know.[29] While this is always part of the picture in a rapidly unfolding scenario such as a pandemic, building trust should be a primary objective of communication.

Messaging should focus on concrete actions and specific time durations—things people can easily process and imagine themselves doing. The cognitive processing required to comprehend the message should be minimal.[29] It should go without saying that messages should be perfectly coordinated across channels to ensure consistency. Motivations behind certain actions and recommendations should always be explained, even if they seem obvious or rudimentary.[29] This helps signal that nothing is being hidden. Communicators should appeal to social norms. This is one of the most powerful psychological behavior-change motivators there is—both the idea that others are already doing the behavior (descriptive norms) and the idea that others believe you should be doing the behavior (injunctive norms).

Government communicators should always try to signal policy coherence, even when dealing with an extraordinary situation such as a pandemic.[30] Policy goals are coherent when they are consistent and political actors behave in ways that are concordant with them. They should also be shared goals with a large number of communities. In the early response to the pandemic in the United States, the administration responded by tying the pandemic to their personal goals of "America first" and sealing the borders. Obviously, focusing on a common goal such as containment that would most likely have spanned across party lines would have created a more coherent foundation for a subsequent set of policies and procedures.[30] Even when containment was no longer possible and the focus should have been on mitigation, Trump would say things like, "We're using the full power of the federal government to defeat the virus," which once again confused people about which policy goal we were pursuing.[30] This made it harder for people to unite around a common cause and to know what actions to take. It also set the government up for a failure of trust because the government promised to contain the pandemic even when it was clearly no longer possible.

We need a better understanding of where communication went wrong, especially during the early days of the pandemic, and what this means in terms of the health of our democracy and the levels of institutional trust in the population. At the most basic level, Trump simply deflected so many questions, that it was at times very difficult to know what he was even talking about. In a July 19, 2020, interview with Chris Wallace of *Fox News*, when asked about the fact that the United States had the seventh highest mortality rate in the world from COVID, Trump deflected the question by arguing that places like Mexico and Brazil are worse and patted himself on the back for having built most of the wall already because that, as he argued, protects us from Mexico.[31] In the same interview, he responded, "nobody knows," to so many questions that it almost became a slogan. His answer to everything was that the World Health Organization got everything wrong and therefore nothing was his fault: "The World Health got a tremendous amount wrong. They basically did whatever China wanted them to and will save now almost $500M a year, which is nice."[31] This is, of course, another kind of deflection that is particularly damaging because it forces people to take sides during a global crisis, which is perverse when considering that unity was probably the number one global need at the moment, and because it directly raises suspicion of the WHO by suggesting they respond only to monetary incentives. In these moments of Trump's "deflections" (and there are many, many of these moments), he creates a rift, a form of defensiveness and a fighting stance, between himself and the interviewer that comes to define the discourse around COVID-19 in the country in general: divided, combative, and ultimately partisan.

Trump and his "crew" regularly used war metaphors when talking about the virus. In an April 13, 2020, press briefing, Trump proclaimed us at "war against the virus."[11] During the same briefing, he said, "Our aggressive strategy to combat the virus is working."[11] Similarly, he commented: "This was a great military and beyond that operation."[11] In an April 2, 2020, briefing, Peter Navarro, Trump's assistant to the president and director of trade and manufacturing policy, added more detail to this picture: "What we have essentially is a nation at war. We have a wartime president standing behind me. The Defense Production Act is one of the most powerful weapons this administration can use to fight the invisible enemy."[13] It is widely recognized that war metaphors to describe an epidemic are unhelpful.[32] They are often another way to deflect attention away from a poor response, and they have the ability to cause stigmatization of those who have the disease and a sense that deaths are "collateral damage," that they were necessary to win the war. It creates an air of aggression and even paternalism, and it gives the president a kind of "wartime" power that might not be appropriate in a response to a pandemic, when a coordinated effort in collaboration with states and federal agencies is needed.

In speaking about actions he had taken to mitigate the virus's spread, Trump always presented himself as clairvoyant and "above" the need to consult with experts and advisors. The decision to ban travel from China early in the pandemic often gets discussed in this vein. In the April 13, 2020, briefing, Trump said: "Not one person had died and I issued the travel ban. . . . I saw what was going on, not so much because I was told, but I saw what was going on."[11] He resists the idea that he followed sage advice to make this decision, but rather that he "saw" himself "what was going on." This insistence that he does not need the consultation of experts, nor to collaborate to formulate a response to the virus, sends a signal to Americans that they should listen only to him. It undermines the authority of state, local, and federal agencies to craft independent responses to the pandemic according to their expertise and what is going on locally. This message of disunity was common in his communication about the virus. He also, not surprisingly, politicized the issue early on, especially by focusing on borders:

> My opposition party wants open borders. This is a case where I'm very glad that my position is I don't want open borders, I want very strong borders, that includes not only on the southern border, our southern border with Mexico, and you could also say our northern border with Canada . . . and I think maybe this is one of the learning points, we learned something about borders . . . a country needs borders to be a great country.[12]

But aside from politicization and undermining authority, there was something else very sinister about the way Trump communicated about the virus, and some of it may have been involuntary. There was a great deal of imprecision and uncertainty in his language without an admission of the real uncertainty involved in the situation. He created discord just by communicating in a way that never settled on an actual answer to anyone's question and that constantly wavered. This display of uncertainty in the absence of an up-front communication of the true uncertainty of the situation was undoubtedly damaging for people who were looking to him for answers (and there were many of those people, at least half the country). For example, in discussing the potential dangers of opening the country up too soon, Trump said: "You talked about couldn't it lead to death, meaning the open up, couldn't it lead to death, and you're right, but y'know what, staying at home leads to death and it's very traumatic for this country, but staying at home, if you look at numbers, leads to a different kind of death perhaps but it leads to death also."[12] Getting off message is common for Trump, but here he does something more damaging: he equivocates and even espouses messages that are typically in conflict with what he is supposed to be promoting. He is supposed to be promoting social distancing, which included mostly staying at home at that point in the pandemic, but instead he starts to argue that staying home could be damaging. At the very least, this is confusing. At the most, it is an underhanded signal to his followers that he does support their eschewal of official public health guidelines.

Reporters regularly picked up on the unevenness of Trump's language. While it might seem subtle, what they were responding to was his refusal to commit to any one tactic or strategy in favor of disease mitigation, not necessarily because he was confused or incompetent, but because he wanted to be able to cater to his base without taking blame for explicitly opposing standard federal public health policy. At a March 14, 2020, press briefing, one reporter called him out on his chameleon ways:

> Your language has changed a bit. You've tweaked it a little bit. Early on, you said there was a low risk for the average American to contract the coronavirus. Recently your language has altered a little bit: you're saying the risk of a serious illness remains low. Can you address why the change? Is the potential of contracting the virus for an average American no longer low, why the change sir?[33]

Trump's carelessness with words could partially be to blame for this change from low risk of contracting the illness to low risk of serious illness.

At the same time, this does seem suspicious, and that suspicion is really what's at the heart of the reporter's question. Trump seemed to have changed his language without announcing that change to the American people. There was never widespread recognition on his part that the risk of contracting the illness was certainly not low. Instead, he slightly altered his language and hoped no one would notice. This phenomenon was basically confirmed in Mike Pence's response: "Everything that we're communicating to the public is based on what is the unanimous opinion of our health experts based upon the information that we have at the time."[33] This response does suggest the potential that a change has occurred, but it still doesn't address the reporter's question—is the risk of *contracting* the illness no longer low? There is no elaboration here for the fact that expert opinion might change over time. There is no room for anticipation of what might happen in the future and how these changes might ultimately confuse and exasperate the American public. Instead, there is a kind of underhanded language game that Trump exploits to cater to his base and downplay the virus at all times. This kind of behavior violates several principles of trustworthy crisis communication, including the need to anticipate how things might unfold and change in the future, the need to stay on message at all times, and the need for transparency.

Although Trump insisted that he was playing nice with state leadership, he often used his press briefings to pick on particular states. During an April 18, 2020, press conference, a reporter asked a question about a member of the coronavirus task force who was organizing protests against stay-at-home orders. Trump responded by going on a short rant about the governor of Michigan, Gretchen Whitmer: "Look, I'm getting along very nicely with the governor of Michigan but she has things 'don't buy paint,' 'don't buy roses,' 'don't buy'—I mean, she's got all these crazy things. There are a lot of protests out there and I just think that some of the governors have gotten carried away." In other words, in his view, it is not a problem to organize an anti-COVID stay-at-home order protest if you believe that the governor has taken the situation "too far." Again, Trump's position is left unclear. The reporter specifically asks about this because Trump wanted us all to be under the impression that he supported social distancing. It was one of the recommendations of his own task force and his own federal government. Yet he refuses to distance himself from protests against it. Once again, he has violated a series of best practices in crisis communication: transparency, clarity of message, and also unity, by turning his back on the leadership of so many states.

When it came to masks, the messaging was a disaster, but this was the case with not only Trump but also his expert advisors, including Birx and Fauci, who faltered on the topic almost just as much. In his April 2, 2020, briefing, Trump said:

> If people wanted to wear them, they can. If people wanted to use scarves, which they have, many people have them, they can. In many cases, the scarf is better, it's thicker, I mean depending on the material it's thicker. But they can do that if they want. Now a recommendation's coming out, we'll see what that recommendation is, but I will say this: they can pretty much decide for themselves.

Trump would repeat this line about scarves many times, which is obviously not scientifically sound, although we did not necessarily establish that until later in the pandemic. He should certainly not have said, "the scarf is better," with no evidence to back this statement up. But we see this equivocation again and this uncertainty about his administration's own recommendations: "Now a recommendation's coming out, we'll see what that recommendation is, but I will say this: they can pretty much decide for themselves." This statement does not establish confidence. It suggests that the administration refuses to take a strong stance on masks and that he may not even know what his own experts think on the topic. While community empowerment is important during a pandemic or any crisis, the idea that the decision is being left up to individual citizens is problematic. The administration does need to display sensitivity and empathy for the experiences and sacrifices of individuals and communities, but it also needs to establish that there are certain scientific recommendations and, if they for some reason cannot mandate them, they should at least communicate in a way that is strong and consistent. Once again, Trump's style of equivocating on the details creates a confusing, free-for-all situation and does not inspire trust in the office of the president or the authority of his experts.

In the early days of the pandemic, although we still needed more information on the efficacy of masking every citizen, Birx did not communicate well on the issue either. In the same April 2, 2020, briefing, she said:

> There is experiential data when you look at communities that have often-times utilized masks in general for personal protection from . . . when they particularly are themselves sick and have used their masks in public and we

looked at the rate of this COVID-19 in those populations and then we're looking at the scientific evidence to bring those 2 pieces together. Let me just say one thing though: the most important thing is the social distancing and washing your hands and we don't want people to get an artificial sense of protection because they're behind a mask because if they're touching things, remember your eyes are not in the mask, so if you're touching things and then touching your eyes you're exposing yourself in the same way. So we don't want people to feel like oh I'm wearing a mask, I'm protected and I'm protecting others.

It's worth parsing this statement a bit. At that point in time, even though it was unclear how effective mass masking would be against COVID-19, she should not have proclaimed that social distancing and washing your hands were more important, because, as it turned out, washing your hands is likely less important than wearing a mask in the case of preventing COVID-19 infection. A good scientist should be able to report on the data we have at the moment without jumping to conclusions about things we might not know. At that point in time, washing hands and social distancing might have *seemed* to be the most important elements of infection response, but we actually did not know enough about masks to say those practices were more important. It was completely unnecessary for her to rank these practices and, especially, to say that masks offer a false sense of security, which may seem logical but was not in fact an evidence-based statement based on empirical behavioral studies. Part of the art of communicating science is to know when to withhold judgment and, in this case, she should have stopped at saying there were experiential data but we were still looking into it.

Even Fauci, who is widely seen as a hero in this story, made some communication missteps. In a January 26, 2022, press briefing, Fauci was asked about whether the Omicron surge was likely to be the last major surge of coronavirus. His answer was long-winded and less than satisfying, as he tried to explain that there has to be a high combination of people with natural immunity and immunity from vaccination in order to see a drop-off in surges of the virus.[34] But he never attempts to give an estimate of the level of immunity needed to reach this stage, and he doesn't share his thoughts on what level of virus circulating in the community would be low enough to avoid future surges. While it is completely understandable that he may not have had reliable numbers for these items, he should have addressed that proactively, sharing that he would like to provide numbers but they were difficult to calculate and the reasons behind that. His and other science communicators' tendency to shy away from transparency around unknown topics, choosing to gloss over them rather than to explicate the uncertainty, can leave people feeling distrustful, as if something is being kept from them.

Fauci also made similar missteps around describing the process for vaccine development. Rather than laying the process out all at once and then reiterating it with consistency, he would often add new layers to the story every time a question about vaccine development came up. In a March 26, 2020, press briefing, an early time in the pandemic when all thoughts were immediately focusing on how to control this with a vaccine, Fauci introduced what seemed like a new wrinkle:

> There's safety associated . . . does the vaccine make you worse? And there are diseases in which you vaccinate someone, they get infected with what you're trying to protect them with and you actually enhance the infection. You can get a good feel for that in animal models. So that's gonna be interspersed at the same time that we're testing we're gonna try and make sure we don't have enhancement. It's the worst possible thing you could do is vaccinate somebody to prevent infection and actually make them worse.[19]

The idea that the vaccine could make you worse had not been broached before, and it would understandably make a lot of Americans uncomfortable. It fed into the idea, used by many anti-vaccine and vaccine-hesitant individuals, that the shot was somehow dangerous. Mentioning that there are diseases in which "when you vaccinate someone, they get infected with what you're trying to protect them with and you actually enhance the infection" was especially problematic. There is a common notion in the vaccine-hesitant world that vaccines cause the illnesses they are purported to prevent. While Dr. Fauci was talking about mere possibilities and a very small number of potential cases, his seeming support of this notion is harmful.

Trump regularly undermined both Fauci and Birx publicly at press briefings and questioned the expertise of important epidemic tools such as infectious disease models. At one point during a March 31, 2020, briefing, after Birx shared that masks were still under consideration, Trump added: "Some people disagree with the masks for various reasons and some people don't but you can wear a scarf, you can do the masks if it makes you feel better, we have no objection to it and some people recommend it." Here we see both the equivocation that is typical of Trump's speech and a form of questioning of what Birx was just saying. Trump gives real consideration to people who "disagree with the masks," saying only that you can wear masks "if it makes you feel better," not that people should pay attention to upcoming recommendations or requirements to wear one.

Similarly, at the same briefing, Fauci shared that effective treatments would take a while to develop, and moments later, Trump added:

> This hydroxychloroquine and azithromycin, which you take with it, maybe, if you want, for the infection, I think some medical workers are doing that, using it maybe, or getting it prescribed perhaps for another use. The word is, some are and some aren't, I think it's not a bad idea to do it, but that's up to the doctors, but there is a theory going around in our country and some other countries people are taking that that work in the hospitals, that work with the patients because there is some evidence, and again it's gonna have to be proven, it's very early, y'know we're rushing this stuff through, this was supposed to take a long time to be approved, and I prevailed the FDA to get it approved immediately on the basis that it was already on the market for a lot of years for another use . . . so we'll see what happens but there is a theory out there that for the medical workers it may work, it may work, and if you take it, y'know it's been out there for a long time.

This statement is obviously problematic, coming on the heels of Fauci's statement that treatments will take time to develop. Trump would go on to pressure scientists working on the vaccine to make sure it came out before the election in November 2020. Again, his speech style is a problem. Even when talking about hydroxychloroquine and azithromycin, two ineffective treatments for COVID-19 that the former president continued to promote, he says, "maybe, if you want" and "using it maybe." He shares that "the word is, some are and some aren't, I think it's not a bad idea to do it, but that's up to the doctors." He suggests that doctors are using it because "there is some evidence, and again it's gonna have to be proven, it's very early." There is no commitment here to providing the American people with a steadfast sense of what treatments are working, if any, and what steps are being taken to bring effective treatments to the many patients who were suffering at that very moment. Trump's statement that "we're rushing this stuff through, this was supposed to take a long time to be approved, and I prevailed the FDA to get it approved immediately on the basis that it was already on the market for a lot of years for another use" also fed the idea that treatments and vaccines for COVID-19 were being "rushed," which gave, and continues to give, many Americans pause over getting the COVID vaccine.

At a time when the country needed clear, consistent, and action-oriented communication, the administration gave them equivocal, vague speech filled with meaningless slogans and problematic notions that the evidence-based scientific process would ultimately not be followed. This was a mistake that was made time and again, not only by the former president himself, but also by some of his top scientific advisors and experts, who were and still are respected in the infectious disease field. To be clear, this was not entirely a partisan issue. The early communications were the most important and the most vulnerable because they set the stage for whether or not Americans were going to trust the government's intervention on this matter. But the Biden administration and the CDC operating under him made numerous communication missteps as well. For one thing, when Biden caught the virus in July 2022, he flouted CDC guidelines by continuing to test himself when the CDC had recommended that people could emerge from isolation 5 days after the onset of symptoms without needing to re-test. The CDC's guidance on masking was confusing, with an initial recommendation that fully vaccinated individuals could stop masking indoors that was reversed several months later. While the reversal itself could not be avoided and made sense in terms of what was learned about the vaccine's ability to prevent against infection and the emergence of new variants, none of this was adequately explained and left many Americans feeling like the CDC didn't know what it was doing. The same could probably be said about boosters. There were multiple booster recommendations that came out over the course of 2021 and 2022 and general confusion about who was eligible when and why they were needed. Many began doubting the efficacy of the vaccine and refusing boosters when they became available because there was never any clear explanation about the natural course of waning immunity and the fact that many vaccines require multiple doses or boosters to be fully effective.

Looking at the comments from some of the early press briefings, it was clear immediately that Americans were losing faith and trust in the process Trump was following. In a YouTube comment on a video of a press briefing that took place on March 31, 2020, one individual wrote: "Your film crew needs training. Either they are intentionally blocking the slides or they haven't figured out how to capture what is important."[35] This actually gets mentioned a lot in the comments on every press briefing, and the fact that the intentions of the administration are being questioned here suggests a deep suspicion of the response effort and of the government itself. In the comments on an April 17, 2020, press briefing, a commenter shared something that sums up a lot of what I have been arguing in this chapter: "Trump is a symptom. What's happened to A,erica [sic] began a generation ago—this, the 'deconstruction of the administrative state' and the pitting of American against American, as tho they were mortal enemies, is the culmination."[19]

Trump's presidency may have been a symptom of a democracy in crisis, but so was the pandemic response both within it and beyond it in Biden's presidency as well. The inability of the Trump administration to provide consistent, clear messaging about the pandemic and the utter confusion about who was in charge and who had the authority to enact emergency procedures and impose restrictions on the American people were egregious failures. At the same time, equivocation about masks, vaccine boosters, and a whole host of other topics during the Biden administration were key factors in the loss of trust in government and public health institutions that many Americans experienced as a result of the response to this pandemic. Quintessentially American issues, such as the problem with federalism and the lack of access to healthcare, especially among marginalized populations, have made the failures here particularly urgent in their signal that the very essence of American democracy might be falling apart. In this way, the response to health emergencies can put the very core of a country to the test. The COVID-19 pandemic certainly did just that, and we collectively failed the test. In her book suggests that we don't have a misinformation problem, we have a trust problem.[36] Issues surrounding science denial that have been around in the United States for over a decade have graduated from being informational issues to being trust issues. At the core of the vast spread of misinformation during and surrounding the pandemic is the shattering of trust in our institutions that is a necessary component of the successful operation of any democracy.[37(p142)] Without that trust, we are teetering very close to a more authoritarian way of life.

Is there a way to restore trust after such an immense failure? While it is difficult, it is not impossible. The Canadian government has invested in infrastructure to build trust and counteract misinformation called Science Up First. A similar initiative, especially with a mandate to study how communications went wrong in response to COVID and how to fix it, is needed in the United States. South Korea's and Taiwan's responses to the pandemic were more successful in part because they built greater institutional capacity for communications. There needs to be a general reckoning that communications are central to public health, rather than being more of an afterthought. As Gounder shared with me, building up the capacity of community health-care workers as trusted messengers is also key to a better response. The situation is not hopeless, but at the moment it is dire. We must continue to understand what the pandemic did to trust and what deeper, preexisting issues it brought to the fore. In the end, we must realize that COVID will never be over—grappling with its legacy is something we can and should continue doing over many years to come.

5

Trust and Well-Being at the Center of Democracy

In the previous chapter, I detailed a complex set of factors that turned our pandemic response into a hopeless failure. When I speak to infectious disease and communications experts about what went wrong, they always have the same initial reaction: "Where do I start?" This is because the roots of the problem run deep into the history of individualism and capitalism in this country, into the anti-safety-net position of many who would greatly benefit from a social safety net, and into the recesses of a slow unraveling of both social and political trust that has left many of us without anything to rely on. In this chapter, I will map these deep histories and explain how we have come to where we are today—sick, despairing, and distrusting.

The loss of trust in the healthcare system is not independent of the loss of trust in other prominent institutions of our democracy—everything is in fact connected. The loss of trust is part of a widespread attack on our social safety net, at the center of which stands healthcare. The crisis of truth and trust in healthcare and other major social institutions may actually be at the root of it all—at the root of widespread distrust in our political institutions, at the root of a crisis of untruth that has spilled over into all areas of information exchange, at the root of a loss of connection with the traditional democratic values of America, and even at the root of the rise to prominence of the far-right extremists who threaten the country's very survival. A general loss of a sense of community and disenfranchisement is also very much part of this story, and this loss of community and social contract is certainly palpable in the healthcare sector and emanates outside it to other social sectors as well.

Experts agree on two matters: one is that there are two types of trust essential to the functioning of democracy. These are trust of the population in government institutions and trust of policymakers in each other.[1(p87)] Some experts add that a certain form of social trust in one another is also essential for the building of the kind of community engagement that encourages participation in democracy. The benefits of social and political trust are numerous, too numerous to name them all here. Some of them most worth mentioning for the purposes of this discussion include: better compliance with emergency measures, such as COVID-19 restrictions (a phenomenon that may have resulted in lower infection rates in societies with greater levels of trust); better performance of the government and fewer bureaucratic "standstills," largely emanating from a sense of responsibility to a populace that expects a certain level of progress; lower levels of corruption; in some cases, greater equity and more social progress in areas such as housing, education, healthcare, and social justice.[2] In the case of the COVID-19 pandemic, trust became an important part of the conversation when researchers discovered something peculiar: the fact that so many higher-income countries had such great levels of mortality from the virus, often higher than many lower-income countries, and the differences could not be explained away by healthcare system features, political factors such as democracy, effectiveness of the state, or social factors such as economic inequality and trust in science.[2] Instead, what seemed especially important in a particular study that characterized some of the potential reasons for this divergence was not only trust, but a particular kind of trust: social trust, or trust in one another. As the authors of the study note, if trust in others in our societies all around the world equaled the high level on display in Denmark, the world would have experienced 40% fewer COVID infections. Similarly, if trust in government around the world had been as high as the high levels in Denmark, the world would have seen 13% fewer infections.[2]

How does the trust relationship work? Why is it so important? And is it really on the decline? These are some of the questions I hope to answer in this chapter, as well as the question about why this trust has been declining in the United States for many decades now. There are, of course, many different types of trust, and thus thinking about it as a monolithic concept is usually a mistake. A society may experience high levels of some types of trust while simultaneously experiencing low levels of other types of trust, which is why it is so important to look at all subtypes when assessing the state of trust in a particular population. The three main types of trust that are most useful to consider are:

1. *Fiduciary trust*, which is a form of trust that occurs between a professional and a non-professional, where there is usually an asymmetry of information. This is the kind of trust we might see between governments and the populace, and, importantly for the subject matter

of this book, the type of trust that exists between healthcare providers
and patients.

2. *Mutual trust*, which refers strictly to the trust between two individuals
who are in some kind of relationship, whether friends, co-workers, or
romantic partners.

3. *Social trust*, where trust is based on expected behaviors in a social setting, and many of these expectations are based on past behaviors.[3] As
we will soon see, this third form of trust, social trust, is particularly important for the story of the breakdown of American trust over the past
30 or so years.

While the loss of trust in political and social institutions may feel like a
recent phenomenon, some believe it can be traced back to the 1990s.[4] There
has been a noticeable decline in trust in government across a variety of nations since that time period, which leads many to believe that it may have
something to do with individual scandals.[4] This might be part of the reason,
but it does not explain the entire phenomenon, especially as it has unfolded
in the past 6 years or so. A lot of the loss of trust, especially in the United
States, is concentrated in politically marginalized groups of people, mostly
unskilled laborers and unemployed individuals, who have not benefited
from the structure of democracy in most societies[4] and have been particularly suffering in the United States, a country with nearly no social safety net.

The financial crisis that unfolded in the United States in 2008 is undoubtedly an important part of the story. The financial crisis led to a loss of faith
in the legitimacy of elites and ultimately in many cases in the democratic
enterprise altogether.[5(p83)] The crisis in 2008 created a pervasive sense in
the United States that the country is governed not for the people but for a
small group of financial elites who in many cases seemed immune to the
consequences of their actions.[5(p83)] These individuals not only were seemingly unaffected by the crisis, but also were seen as passing their massive
costs along to everyone else.[5(p83)] The financial crisis may even have paved
the way for populism, a movement that reared its ugly head most obviously
during Trump's presidency.[5(p82)] Historian Geoffrey Hosking has suggested
that the current populist movement arises from a breakdown in the alliance
between democracy and capitalism and argues that this has happened in
four stages over the past several decades, starting with inflation in the 1970s,
public indebtedness in the 1980s, private debt in the 1990s and early 2000s,
and a terminal crisis beginning in 2008.[5(p82)] According to him, democracy

and the U.S. economy are in their final years, struggling to survive as joint, interdependent entities. The world we once knew, in which we enjoyed an array of financial opportunities and democratic freedoms, is coming to an end, and the financial crisis of 2008 played no small part in this erosion of American society.

The 2008 financial crisis brought to the fore many of the ways in which our society was (and still is) functioning in a manner that is fundamentally unequal. Increasing economic inequality is a major factor in growing distrust of government institutions, with people in rural communities in the United States viewing the mostly urban elites as responsible for their misfortune. As a result, they favor limited government action, even though a greater degree of government involvement in a better social safety net might actually be helpful for people dealing with economic distress.[6] Lack of economic mobility is also a major factor in public trust, and this has a largely comparative component to it as well, as people compare their lot in life and their inability to climb the ladder to people who have reached the top and seem to have all the advantages of government and democratic society conferred upon them.[6] But perhaps most important is the perception of fairness. There is a strong relationship between trust and the perception of fairness. In fact, Angus Deaton notes that perception is probably even more important than reality in the development and maintenance of trust in public institutions.[6] The sense of how fair the distribution of wealth is across a society is a centerpiece of public trust in government. Indeed, trust in government and perceptions of fairness track each other almost identically over the past half century.[6]

Just how bad is the trust "crisis" in American society? Different people tend to cite different numbers, but a 2022 Pew poll found that 20% of Americans said they trust Washington to do the right thing most or all of the time; 8% said they thought the government was responsive to the needs of the American people. About a quarter of Americans say the government has done a good job of dealing with immigration and getting people out of poverty; 60% or more of Americans say the government should have a large part in addressing 11 of 12 policy areas, including access to healthcare and protecting the environment; 52% say the government should play a major role in helping people out of poverty. Relatively few think the government is responsive to citizens' needs, that they use the taxpayer money well, or that they respond well to new challenges. Six in 10 say the notion that it favors some people over others describes the federal government extremely or very well—this is not a very partisan response. The same is true of whether people think the government can handle new challenges well—across party lines, people think it can't. And 71% of Americans think the government is holding information back from the general public. A majority (53%) think the government should do more to deal with major societal problems. State and local governments are generally viewed more favorably than the federal government.[7]

There are some particularly notable findings here. It probably surprises no one that only 20% of Americans trust Washington to do the right thing. In an era of extreme political infighting and a general inability to get anything done, one might almost wonder why even 20% of people maintain so much faith in the federal government. What is most telling here for our purposes is the sense people have that the government is not doing enough to address societal needs and the conviction that it should be doing more. Despite accusations that Americans think private enterprises should deal with all societal issues and that they are selfish and don't care about societal problems, a 53% majority of Americans believe the American government should do more to deal with societal problems. The 60% who agreed that the government should do more in a majority of listed societal areas named healthcare as a major area in need of more federal government attention. All of these findings pertain to the idea that trust in government is at least somewhat moderated by the sense that government action is effective. But what's even more important here is the fact that distrust of the government arises in part from the specific idea that the government is not doing enough to deal with societal harms. The general collapse and inefficacy of our healthcare system is certainly one of these harms, and its general decay is something that most likely has caused a decline in trust in the very institutions that are supposed to be governing it.

Important for this discussion and for our understanding of so-called deaths of despair, which will be examined below, is the fact that social status interacts in profound ways with trust in the government. Trust in government is almost always higher among more highly educated and wealthier individuals.[8] This is generally true in the United States and other high-income countries. People's personal financial concerns, perception of relatively lower status in society, and a pervasive feeling of being left behind by government decision-making all negatively impact levels of trust in government.[8] Interestingly and importantly, perceived social status impacts trust more than actual level of income or education level, suggesting that this trust issue is very much subjective and can be a result of perception in some cases, rather than reality.[8]

Despite the common refrain that Americans hate government regulation, they are actually much more likely to say that they would like more regulation rather than less.[9] Even when Americans say they don't trust the government, they will often simultaneously divulge that they'd like the government to do more in their lives.[9] This shouldn't be surprising, as there really is an implicit contract between the state and citizens that the state will secure the well-being of the populace, including helping to provide economic security and social services, such as healthcare and education.[10]

Trust in the government is also much more partisan now than it used to be, which also should not be surprising. Americans are now much more likely to respond that they trust the government if their particular party is in power, and much less likely to respond that they trust the government if it is not.[11] Still, everyone agrees that the government, whether run by Democrats or Republicans, should absolutely do more to fix social problems.[11] We should also recognize that growing distrust in the government is not completely inadvertent—politicians, especially on the right, have tried to promote it by arguing that institutions they do not control are somehow corrupt and untrustworthy.[12] There has even been a decline over the years of the sort of "big government" liberalism seen in the FDR era. In the 1960s and 1970s, liberals fought the government primarily around issues relating to the environment that created a strain of anti-government sentiment on the left.[12] It might be argued that the anti-vaccine movement arose from this strain of anti-government liberalism. Some scholars have argued that the Bill Clinton era was the real turning point in the history of governmental manipulation of the truth, with Newt Gingrich emerging as the primary strategist.[12] So the truth crisis we face now is not entirely new, although it is accompanied by soaring levels of despair and human destruction, which I will discuss more at length in the next section. In the meantime, it is also important to note that just because this crisis of truth and trust might seem to be a game waged by political elites, citizens are by no means unwitting pawns and by all means have had a part to play, and they continue to play a role in shaping and disseminating the "truth."[12]

Deaths of Despair: The Crisis of Healthcare as a Crisis of the Middle Class

In his book *Dying of Whiteness*, Jonathan Metzl tells a horrifying story of a 41-year-old White taxi driver in Tennessee who refused treatment for life-threatening inflammation of his liver. The Tennessee legislature had not taken up any part of the Affordable Care Act and had not expanded Medicaid. In Kentucky, however, the man could receive treatment for an affordable amount. As he became more and more ill, he stood by his conviction that he did not want the government involved in his healthcare. As he put it:

"No way I want my tax dollars paying for Mexicans or welfare queens." Even more forcefully, he told Metzl: "Ain't no way I would ever support Obamacare or sign up for it. I would rather die." The man went on to die of a treatable condition all because he did not want the government to pay for his treatment, in case supporting this kind of government involvement would mean giving his hard-earned money to the "Mexicans" and the "welfare queens."[13(p189)] This example is a good entry point into a discussion about the partisan nature of healthcare and the complexities associated with Americans' feelings about the healthcare system.

But first a bit more on the complex nature of trust to set us up for a discussion about the relationship between healthcare access and governmental trust. Many people think that trust in the government is securely tied to its performance, but this is not always the case.[14(p6)] This also suggests that trust increases with knowledge of how the government is performing, but a lot of trust is based on what are called identification-based factors, which have more to do with shared value than actual performance.[14(p6)] Some even argue that pure knowledge-based trust is really just "confidence" and that true trust depends on at least some identification and values-based factors.[14(p6)] There is also a distinction to be drawn between "rational" or "instrumental" trust, which is something like "I trust you because I believe it is not in your interest to betray me" versus "social" trust," which is more like "I trust you because I believe you will not betray me even if it is in your best interest to do so."[14(p20)] These distinctions are important because they suggest that trust is subject to subjective assessments and values-based judgments, rather than simply being a product of having been betrayed or losing faith in an entity for some reason.

If trust is at least partially about values, it would make sense that people who feel philosophically that the government should take care of their health and well-being might lose trust when they see that is not what happens. This line of thinking and making values-based judgments is also what causes trust to fall when societies are viewed as inequitable. In one survey of a large sample of Americans, 50% of people said they thought the government helps wealthy people the most.[15] A minority (around 37%–39%) said they felt the government helped people "like me" or "my community."[15] This sense of abandonment, especially the idea that the society is inequitable, is a major driver of distrust.

It should be no surprise, then, that perceptions of inequity in the health-care system would lead many to a place of despair. The ill health of the healthcare system is in fact at the center of an epidemic of "deaths of despair," according to Case and Deaton in their landmark book *Deaths of Despair and the Future of Capitalism.* The term "deaths of despair" refers to the growing phenomenon of deaths from overdose and suicide that has characterized a loss of life expectancy in the White working class over the course of the past 2 decades. For Case and Deaton, it is not simply a matter of blaming the economy. While it's true that economic distress can cause despair, this epidemic, in their view, did not originate there. Instead, it originated with major failures of the healthcare system to regulate itself. While the opioid scandal represents the most obvious example of a major failure of the healthcare system to protect its constituents from a dangerous class of drugs, as Case and Deaton argue, "[t]he problems with the healthcare industry go far beyond the opioid scandal."[16(p10)] Instead, they say: "The US spends huge sums of money for some of the worst health outcomes in the Western world. We will argue that the industry is a cancer at the heart of the economy, one that has widely metastasized, bringing down wages, destroying good jobs, and making it harder and harder for state and federal governments to afford what their constituents need."[16(p10)] The very nature of our healthcare system, with its extreme costs and the absolute failure of our health insurance system to adequately cover people who need it, has literally driven people to despair. Healthcare has bankrupted individuals, states, and the federal government and has left people desperate, sick, and, indeed, in despair. Without understanding the healthcare system, according to Case and Deaton, we cannot understand what is happening to our economy, our collective well-being, and even our society writ large. The betrayal of the government to care for its people on such a basic level as securing their health and well-being has led to increasing alienation of citizens from the centers of power and increased willingness to believe in fringe ideas and alternative political viewpoints. The government has abandoned us, and we have abandoned the government.

Deaths of despair are very much a phenomenon of a lower socioeconomic White population without a college education. For many of them, three institutions in the United States have primarily failed them: the healthcare system, which in many instances has not adequately taken care of their pain

and has left them in debt and without access to high-quality care; the education system, which turns out not to be a meritocracy; and the labor market,
which has left many of them unemployed, in their view often directly an
effect of immigration and employment of foreign laborers for smaller
incomes. In 2019, only about half of Americans thought that institutions of
higher education were having a positive effect on American society; 59% of
Republicans, which is the party that has become increasingly less educated,
thought institutions of higher education were having a negative impact on
American society.[16(p55)] An unequal meritocracy, in which some are clear
"winners" and some are clear "losers," can lead to a horrible sense of resentment. These meritocracies are unequal in many cases because there has been
some form of cheating, as Case and Deaton point out: "When meritocracies
are unequal, as is the case in the US today, with vast rewards for successfully
identified merit—passing exams, promotions, making partner, speculating
successfully, or getting elected—the rewards are paid not only for ability
and virtue but also for cheating and for abandoning long-held ethical
constraints that are seen as impediments to success."[16(p55)] The standards of
public behavior are low, and members of the elite are seen as corrupt by the
"outgroup." As discussed earlier, this kind of inequality is also characteristic
of the U.S. healthcare system.

White Americans below a certain income level who lack a college education are also more likely to report being in chronic pain than any other
group of people in the United States.[16(pp86–87)] Case and Deaton even report that "[t]he fraction of people in an area who voted for Donald Trump
in 2016 is also strongly correlated with the fraction in pain."[16(pp86–87)] There
is therefore a strong correlation among poverty and unemployment, lack
of a college education, identifying as White, supporting Trump, and being
in chronic pain. The profile of a White American living somewhere in the
middle of the country wearing a MAGA hat is also more likely to be the profile of someone who is in constant and likely significant pain—significant
enough to repeatedly seek out opioids. The reasons for this inequality in who
experiences chronic pain in this country are not entirely clear. It could be
that people in these communities have poorer healthcare, which may have
increased the risk of developing pain in the first place, or it could be related
to lack of access to good healthcare to deal with the pain before it becomes
chronic, or perhaps both of these factors are at play. What is clear is that the
opioid epidemic and the soaring levels of despair associated with it originate
once again in a system that is unequal, that allows some people immediate

access to the highest-quality care, for a price, and leaves others wallowing in the depths of addiction, psychological pain, and a high dose of resentment. This has not boded well for the country's ability to unite around common challenges such as the COVID-19 pandemic, and has left many feeling like our broken system needs a savior—preferably a savior who does not represent the institutions that have already failed them.

American healthcare has been a serious drain on our capitalist system, but it also represents it in some interesting ways. As Case and Deaton put it, the healthcare system utilizes "market power to bring about upward redistribution, from a large number of people with little, to a smaller number with a great deal." Who benefits from this system? Certainly rich people who are stockholders in American healthcare companies, including pharmaceutical and biotech companies as well as insurance companies, but also members of the educated elite who hold stock indirectly via retirement funds. As Case and Deaton argue, "this process, run out over half a century, has slowly eaten away at the foundations of working-class life, high wages and good jobs, and has been central in causing deaths of despair. The opioid story fits with this more general theme but is much more flagrant, because it is rare that corporations can so directly benefit from death."[16(pp126–127)] The healthcare system, and its operation as an important lever of capitalism in our highly unequal society, is killing people by the tens of thousands.

This growing sense of economic inequality probably started sometime after the 1970s. From the end of World War II until the 1970s, economic growth was good and it was also well distributed.[16(p149)] This growth lifted people of all incomes and education levels. After the 1970s, growth both slowed and became increasingly unequal.[16(p149)] This kind of growth has probably been more unequal in the United States than in other high-income countries and may in some ways have contributed to the more severe trust crisis we have in this country than is evident in many Western European countries that seem similar to us otherwise. For one thing, we have severe racial inequalities in this country that have developed under the shadow of slavery. The stark history of racial divides in this country is still at play in the complex relationship between the growth in African American well-being and prosperity over the decades of the latter half of the 20th century and into the 21st century and the ways in which this has impacted the attitudes of uneducated, White, mostly rural Americans who have perceived that they are somehow losing their jobs to Black and immigrant workers.[16(pp186–187)] Case and Deaton have been rightly criticized for underplaying the continued economic disadvantages experienced by non-White minority populations in the United States. A more recent editorial in the *Lancet* has suggested that their argument and the subsequent scholarship on this topic have not taken into account the very sharp rise in mortality among indigenous populations in the United States, especially since the pandemic began in 2020.[17] To be clear, what I am highlighting in this chapter is a White working-class *perception* that mostly Black populations have gained ground, while they have lost their jobs and have withered economically and socially. The perception creates a lot of the attitudes and behaviors that I am interested in here, including mistrust of the government and health authorities. I am not, however, discounting the fact that many, if not most, of these feelings come from a place of deeply situated racism.

The other story about White working-class "decline," real or perceived, and the slippery slope into despair has to do with social protection, or rather the lack of it. European countries have much more extensive safety nets that the American system, and citizens there are much more dependent on the government than on the private sector, the polar opposite of the structures in place in the United States.[16(pp186–187)] The campaign financing and extensive corporate lobbying that drives American politics are also part of the story. Healthcare companies, including pharmaceutical companies, have a lot of money and a powerful lobby in Washington.[16(pp186–187)] This kind of capital-dependent governmental system allows companies that often do not work in the best interest of Americans' health and well-being to often have a larger say in political matters than the people themselves. The lack of a social safety net creates a crisis of access and treatment that has certainly led people to feel abandoned, as has been argued elsewhere in this chapter and in this book. Many members of the working class have as a result turned their backs on the government and instead embraced free-market capitalism, which might seem like an odd choice given the fact that many of their lives have been ruined by corporate America's destruction of both fair working conditions and the natural environment. And yet trusting the government, which has done basically nothing to protect them, feels like a fool's errand. In my interviews, I heard from a lot of people with working-class jobs who had been laid off. Most of the distrust of the system they developed occurred after they lost their jobs. While it is possible that they just had more time on their hands to root around the Internet, they all expressed a strong sense of betrayal and disillusionment that was never directed at corporations but got channeled toward government authorities, especially during the pandemic.

In addition to these issues surrounding access and undue corporate influence is the very real issue of cost. Case and Deaton argue that this is the most
important driver of deaths of despair in the United States. They argue that
healthcare costs are an impossible drag on the American economy, pushing
down wages, reducing the number of good jobs, and leaving little money for
infrastructure and a whole array of other public goods and provisions that
might be provided by federal or state governments. In their view, while it
is true that automation and globalization are impacting working-class jobs,
the greater threat is coming from the astronomical costs of the healthcare
system.[16(pp186–187)] [51] As they argue, "The truth is that these horrors are
happening not *in spite of* the American healthcare system but *because of*
it."[16(pp186–187)]

American institutions, therefore, are at the center of American problems,
including the fall into despair of the White working class. This has not only
caused deaths of despair, but in some cases also has contributed to political
and ideological extremism and hatred. While globalization and automation
are still an important part of this story, it is the fabric of uniquely American
institutions, including most essentially the healthcare system, that has led
to these tragic consequences.[16(pp222–223)] Why is the social safety net in the
United States basically nonexistent, when this same kind of supportive structure is so present in our European counterparts? The question is obviously
complex. Many cite American individualism as the answer—America has a
history of emphasizing the individual that extends all the way back to the
founding fathers, and there is no way that such a fiercely individualistic culture would ever support the government's involvement in supporting people
who struggle financially or otherwise. No individualistic American would
ever want to pay into such a set of programs. Some part of this is probably
true, but Case and Deaton argue that we should pay more attention to issues
around race and immigration as well. People are less willing to participate
in programs that benefit people who do not look like them. Even now, state-
level benefits are less generous in states with larger Black populations.[16(p224)]

Despite this resistance to government involvement in what many
Americans believe should be private and individual affairs, a 2021 Pew poll
found that 64% of Americans believe it is the government's responsibility to
provide healthcare to its citizens.[18] This conviction largely cuts across party
lines. At the same time, barely one-fifth of American citizens believe the government is doing a good job at addressing health, education, and the environment.[11] And while citizens want the government to take care of their

health, they still don't trust the government or affiliated health agencies.[19,20] In Chapter 4, I discussed the fact that fostering citizens' basic health and well-being is one of the most fundamental aspects of a well-functioning, democratic governing body. Most Americans seem to have internalized this idea, with accompanying expectations that the government meet their basic needs, even if there are heated partisan arguments about exactly how the government should be involved. A minority of people feel strongly that the government has no part to play in helping citizens secure a basic degree of health and well-being. When we think about how extensively the American government has failed to look after its citizens in this way, leaving people uninsured, sick, and in some cases, plunging into the depths of despair, it is no wonder that trust in the government is waning. The shiny gloss on New Deal–era healthcare reforms has fully faded, and we are left with nothing but a broken system and a series of shattered promises.

The Long View: Crises of Trust That Preceded Trump

When I discuss the topic of this book with people, many people's thoughts immediately go to Trump and his political followers. While it is true that Trump-era deceptions led to and coincided with record-high levels of distrust in traditional forms of American government, in almost all our social and political institutions, and in all official forms of communication to the point that people were believing outright lies, the decline in trust in the United States did not start with Trump. If we are to understand how basic government information became so contentious during Trump's reign, we must explore what came before him, and we need to go back several decades to do that successfully.

The 2008 financial crisis is an important moment that needs to be considered in any analysis of trust in our institutions in this country, including healthcare institutions. In traditional theories of capitalism, theorists such as Adam Smith held that trust in financial institutions is not that important because markets are self-correcting and always functional. This turns out to be extremely far from the truth. If the 2008 financial crisis taught us anything, it taught us that traditional economic theories, in which the market took care of itself, were dead and that trust was in fact paramount.[5] In the aftermath of the crisis, banks no longer trusted each other, and this has at times led to dysfunction in our financial institutions.[5(p85)] The realization in the general population that the world's 1% lived in an untouchable state of luxury that largely disregarded the rest of society was a brutal reckoning. Ongoing revelations, such as the 2016 uncovering of the Panama papers, have simply continued to sow distrust and discord, especially between the working class and the top 1% of society.[5(p89)] These kinds of revelations showed the rest of the world that the extremely wealthy were essentially able to hide their wealth without having to pay taxes, while the rest of us paid a sizable portion of our much smaller incomes back to the government. This moment stoked the fires for the eventual rise of populism.

At the same time, a form of "gig" economy has arisen that has left workers feeling abandoned and abused. In the 1930s, even as there was a major clash between national trust and the international economy, workers could take comfort in a form of social solidarity they had with one another.[5(pp101–102)] Now everyone is simply a nameless, faceless, and largely interchangeable work product, and the desire for a new face to trust in, one that is preferably outside the existing establishment, has become ever more potent.

As much as this moment of relinquished institutional trust and dismay over the changing demographics of our society feels unique, this is not the first time this has happened in this country. Andrew Jackson's presidency, from 1829 to 1837, has historically been considered anti-aristocratic and a time when restless workers became a political force. It was a time of dramatically high rates of immigration and fast-paced economic change, coinciding with the rise of manufacturing.[21(p55)] Jackson was known for railing against the political "establishment," trying at every turn to obliterate what he felt was the overwhelming power of the existing federal government.[21(p57)] In his words, he wanted everything to come back to a form of "primitive simplicity and purity," and in his vision the "machinery" of Washington would be "so simple and economical as scarcely to be felt."[21(p57)] Talk about "purity" in light of record high rates of immigration is especially ominous. Not surprisingly, Jackson's rhetoric appealed to "restless" workers who railed against the policies of a federal government that was allowing their country to be "taken away" from them. New economic opportunities would not be lost to immigrants under any circumstances. The answer was to pour support behind a man who promised a better way.

In the presidency of Andrew Johnson in the post–Civil War era, we can see strong reflections of the principles of Jackson's presidency as well. In a presaging of the modern-day fight over welfare, Johnson turned his supporters against the Freedman Bureau, which he thought was just a "giveaway" to Black Americans.[21(p105)] In his view, the federal government should operate in a "minimal" manner, and the principles of individualism and property rights were to be sanctified.[21(p105)] Welfare-giving bureaucracies were all, in his mind, radical structures to be derided and demoted.[21(p105)]

As Greg Grandin outlines in his book *The End of the Myth*, the "Frontier Thesis" was a form of founding principle in the United States based on rugged individualism and a distaste for centralized federal power. If this was the prevailing theory throughout the era of the founding fathers, through the Civil War and Reconstruction period, and up through World War I, the New Deal era cast itself as the antithesis to these ideas. The New Deal offered a sharp critique of laissez-faire individualism and espoused the idea that freedom in a complex society did require government intervention. After all, as FDR said, "necessitous men are not free."[21(p179)]

Our modern moment can be seen as a counterpart to the New Deal era in many ways, a time when capitalism reigns, suspicion of government programming and aid is rampant, and a focus on individual will and freedom, often at the expense of the well-being and even survival of others, is palpable at every turn. Clearly, our current predicament did not arise in the past several years or exclusively as a result of a former president who treated facts as suggestions. In his new book, *The Destructionists: Inside the Twenty-Five Year Crack-Up of the Republican Party*, Dana Milbank argues that the ills of the present moment are not new, but emerged as a result of a 25-year struggle with the truth on the part of the Republic Party.[22] In his view, this casual relationship with the truth started around the time that Clinton assumed the presidency and had its strongest advocate in Gingrich. The first set of lies was the suggestion that Clinton's top aide, Vince Foster, who tragically died by suicide, was actually murdered by the Clintons. An investigation, which dragged on for several years, was actually opened up as a result of this conspiracy theory. In the end, the Republicans dropped the theory when the investigation found no evidence for foul play. Today, that conspiracy theory would probably have continued to spread with gusto. Milbank still brands this event a "prototype" for the kind of conspiratorial thinking and utilization of government resources to chase partisan, often harmful, claims that very much characterizes this moment.[22] As Milbank argues, Trump often brought conspiracy theories to the fore, but did not necessarily create them anew.[22(p211)]

A Loss of Connection and the Rise of the Alt-Right

All of this lying and cheating cannot be good for citizens' trust in the government. And while those who believe the lies may be seen as finding a sense of "belonging" within the confines of the lying party, there is an important way in which the failure of the American social safety net over the past several decades has left certain citizens particularly stranded, and their loss of a sense of home and safety has led to the increased appeal of far-right ideologies and authoritarianism.

An important part of overall trust in the government and an important indicator of civic participation is something called "social capital," which refers to "social connections, networks and interpersonal trust that occur in communities."[14(p25)] Changes in social capital can have a substantive effect on trust in government bodies. A substantial loss in social connections, networks, and connection to local communities can lead to loss in overall trust in society and the government writ large. When citizens become disengaged from civic life and experience a lack of social reciprocity, they struggle to trust governing institutions.[14(p25)]

In the United States, levels of alienation from the government and a sense of being abandoned and not looked after are very high. While almost every other industrial nation has pursued free trade policies similar to those in the United States, including some combination of outsourcing, privatization, and financial liberalization, no other industrialized nation has experienced the kind of alienation, inequality, public health crises, and violence that are now such a central part of the American experience. As Grandin argues, the post-Vietnam era saw an "assault" on our social institutions, especially unions and public services. As Reagan told his right-wing activists working to unravel the New Deal: "You're out there on the frontier of freedom."[21(p271)] And so the end of the New Deal era and the rebirth of the Frontier mentality was upon us.

In her in-depth study of the emerging far right, Arlie Hochschild paints a portrait of a group of people repeatedly wronged and harmed by industry but clinging to a faith in its value and a potent eschewal of all things "government." At the center of this moral crisis is a feeling of having been robbed in some way of their country, being bereft of their land, their place in the world, and their honor.[23(p47)] Working-class America feels over-regulated by the government, and yet in reality the government does not do enough to stop the serious damage to health, well-being, and the natural environment wrought by industry. This probably feeds into a sense of powerlessness.[23(p51)] There is a vast amount of environmental damage in places such as Louisiana, for example, and politicians have done little to clean it up.[23(p47)]

Counterintuitvely, despite the havoc wrought by industry, working-class people in places highly affected, such as Louisiana, do not feel warmly toward government regulation. In fact, if you live in a highly polluted state, you are much more likely to believe that the people worry too much about pollution, that the government is doing more than enough about it, and you are more likely to be a Republican.[23(p79)] This is the sort of set of attitudes that leads Hochschild to dub the situation in rural, right-leaning states the "Great Paradox." The idea is that despite being repeatedly wronged by industry, people in these states are still largely opposed to more government regulation and generally trust industry far more than they trust the government.

Beneath the Great Paradox is a narrative that Hochschild calls the "deep story." The "deep story" goes something like this: people want to live the American Dream but for various reasons feel they have been held back. As a result, they become increasingly frustrated and especially angry at the government, on which they place most of the blame for their lack of upward mobility.[23(p149)] Interestingly, as Hochschild points out, a lot of the dissatisfaction expressed by the right about a failure to achieve the American Dream is not that different from left-leaning Occupy-type protests, where the issue is fairness (and the lack of it). The difference is that the right-leaning population has split everyone up into the "takers" and the "makers," where the "takers" are those who rely on the welfare system and the "makers" are those who work. In their view, the unfairness comes from an over-reliance on government assistance, as opposed to the locus of unfairness in the left-leaning Occupy movement, which centers around industry and the wealthiest of the wealthy.[23(p149)] While the structure is similar, the center focus of injustice is on the public sector on the right and the private sector on the left.

In this narrative, what ultimately set the stage for Trump? In Hochschild's vision, a lot of the fodder for the Trump-era right-wing surge ultimately came from the Tea Party. In her telling, Tea Party supporters felt on shaky economic ground starting in the 1980s. In addition, they felt culturally marginalized, with their traditional views about marriage, abortion, gender roles, and gay rights becoming less and less popular, as well as being opposed to new federal government laws and policies (although much of this has reversed in recent years).[23(p221)] They felt, and in many ways still feel, part of a demographic decline of "White Christians."[23(p221)] As Hochschild points out, this represented a real change from the way people dealt with the economic downturn in the 1930s, in which people placed their faith in the public sector. In the economic downturn that really began and continued from the early 2000s, partially as a result of increasing globalization and automation, people have placed their faith in capitalism.[23(p229)]

There is an overwhelming feeling, in Hochschild's work as well as in the work of several other scholars, that fundamentalist, far-right White Americans, many of whom live in the rural South, have been wronged by both the government and industry and are, in many ways, victims of multiple systems at work, but that they still somehow continue to vote against their own interests.[24] Oil became the new "cotton" of the South, and, as Hochschild argues, cotton was taken away from Southerners in a manner that felt damaging to their pride and personhood. When "Big Oil" came along, many White Southerners felt they had something to be proud of again, even though this nameless, faceless industry wound up polluting their land and leaving many of them sick and injured.[23(p210)] White Southerners are really victims of both industry and the government to a certain extent. Although, as a concept, additional government intervention would ultimately help them, the reality is that the government has also failed White Southerners by not providing them with enough of a social safety net, especially in times of economic turmoil that were completely out of citizens' control. Politicians often play into this feeling of victimhood, even though they are part of the problem.[23(p231)] In her acclaimed book *Caste*, Isabel Wilkerson argues that by voting against the government, right-wing White Americans might be *actually* voting against their own interests, but maintaining the caste system creates the illusion that they are voting in their own interests:

> Caste gives insights, too, into the Democrats' wistful yearning for white working-class voters that they believe should respond in higher numbers to their kitchen table appeals. Why, some people on the left kept asking, why, oh, why, were these people voting against their own interests? The questioners on the left were unseeing and yet so certain. What they had not considered was that the people voting this way were, in fact, voting their interests. Maintaining the caste system as it had always been was in their interest. And some were willing to accept short-term discomfort, forgo health insurance, risk contamination of the water and air, and even die to protect their long-term interest in the hierarchy as they had known it.[13(p327)]

In other words, right-wing White Americans are willing to destroy the government and all it has to offer them, in terms of a safety net and protection of the very air they breathe and water they drink, in order to maintain a world order that keeps people of color, especially Black people, beneath them. The maintenance of hierarchy trumps all other concerns, in Wilkerson's telling.

I think this account is absolutely true, but it should be combined with the story told by Hochschild and others about the increasing isolation and alienation of working-class White Americans. Hochschild discusses the ills wrought by industry on the working class, but she also spends a lot of time detailing the various ways in which the government has abandoned, and in some cases even exploited, its members. This dovetails well with Case and Deaton's argument about the rise of deaths of despair. In many cases feeling divorced from the deep histories of both land and country, stranded without a social safety net, without health insurance or any other kind of government assistance, and without reassurance that the land around them will not be destroyed or that dangerous chemicals will not be released into the air and water, these people are literally dying in greater numbers despite decades of advancement in healthcare and medical science. Their answer to this devastating turn of events? Dig their heels in, reject the government altogether, and fight for a new order, one in which nostalgia about the past is satisfied by demanding the ruin of classes and races that make the world look different than it did when they were more secure and healthier.

Why does trust in government matter? There are numerous reasons, including increased willingness to participate in civic activities such as voting and the development of a sense of community that helps people care for one another. The COVID crisis showed us a very particular way in which trust in government matters. An important study found that overall trust in government was more important than other factors, such as the capacity of the healthcare system, when mitigating the spread of COVID.[25]

As discussed earlier, trust in others, or certain forms of social trust, has also been found to be incredibly important in the context of improving pandemic outcomes.[25] In fact, vaccine hesitancy, which has been a major barrier to a successful pandemic response in the United States, represents a form of break in the social contract—the idea that you cannot rely on people to take an action that will help others is a problem in any society. When governments cut social programs, it erodes trust in the government to be certain, but also, importantly, it can chip away at any existing sense of community, solidarity, and citizenship.[26] People become more isolated, alienated, and less concerned about what happens to those around them. They take less responsibility for doing everything they can to preserve the lives of their community members. Of course a form of rugged individualism has been a part of the American ethos since the beginning. But the kind of community alienation, the kind of extreme isolation that can ultimately drive people to despair—this ailment is somewhat new, and it is a serious scourge of our time. The kind of universal social programming that marked the era of the Great Society creates a sense of individual flourishing, but it also creates a sense of community flourishing as well.[27] This is what we are now missing.

Throughout this book, we have followed the journey of our contemporary moment from mistrust in healthcare to conspiracy theories and to the failure of our entire governmental and societal operation to support our population in ways that would preserve trust and encourage participation in important social directives such as getting vaccinated against a pandemic disease. We have seen how contemporary loss of community and a social safety net has driven some to despair and others to extremism. We have also seen how the system itself has made us distrust it, with lack of access to healthcare in many cases causing conspiracy beliefs about health and medicine. Now that I have mapped what certainly at the moment feels like a hopeless calamity, it is time to get a better understanding of what can and should be done about it. Repairing decades of government neglect is not an easy feat, but there are things to be done to radically improve our information ecosystem, to fortify people against the impact of extremist messages, and to build back a sense of community where alienation and despair reign. In the next chapter, I will attempt to do just that.

6

Symptoms of Mistrust and What to Do About Them

In an interview I conducted in the winter of 2023, a young woman from the Boston area told me her mother had been pulled into a deep sense of medical mistrust, which ultimately probably caused her death, from believing misinformation from her chiropractor. This trajectory is quite common: engagement with medical misinformation may eventually lead to a kind of deep-seated distrust of the entire healthcare system. I have spent much of this book expounding on some of the major structural and systemic problems that the healthcare system and other social systems face and that have increased medical mistrust and belief in conspiracy theories. In this chapter, I want to offer a few potential solutions. I will focus much of my attention here on misinformation, as it is both a common gateway to mistrust and also represents a "symptom" of a society in which overall trust has declined. I will also discuss what exists in the literature about rebuilding trust in our most central social institutions. Lest the reader despair at all that we still do not know about rebuilding trust and quelling the rise of misinformation, it is worth noting that these are still very active fields of study with evidence on new interventions coming out almost daily. I will cover what is most up to date at the time of this writing.

While many scholars and public intellectuals agree that trust in our social and political institutions in the United States is waning, there is a dearth of evidence on what would work to improve the situation. Nonetheless, there are studies that might prove useful in their ability to isolate some of the reasons why trust has fallen (and continues to fall). A Pew study from 2019, albeit before the pandemic in which the situation got worse, is instructive in providing insight into some of the key reasons why trust, especially in the government, is waning. Americans on the whole agree that trust in the government is declining. There is a sense of increased individualism and a broken political system that spawns suspicion and cynicism.[1] Perhaps surprisingly, and somewhat encouraging, is the fact that a vast majority of

Americans believe both trust in government and trust in each other (sometimes referred to as social trust) can improve.[1] Some findings were surprising, most notably that only 36% of people agreed that the decline in trust is due to poor government performance. Common wisdom tends to be that in times of good perceived government performance, trust will be high, and in times of poor perceived government performance, trust will decline. However, this study suggests that performance is not the main ingredient in determining governmental trust. Instead, there are other, potentially more important, factors, including the state of the political system and the health of the information ecosystem. In some cases, then, the government can perform well, in that it does its job and responds to citizen needs promptly, but distrust might still be high.

In this study, there were some interesting demographic characteristics of note. For example, 49% of Americans believed other people are less reliable than they used to be, but those who believed this were more likely to be Republicans, to make $30K or less per year, and to lack a college education.[1] The study also broke people into three groups based on their levels of trust: "high-trust" individuals, "medium-trust" individuals, and "low-trust" individuals. These cutoffs were determined by presenting scenarios to people and seeing how often they chose "pro-trust" responses. The study found that 22% of Americans are "high trusters," with White people being twice as likely as Black and Latinx individuals to fall into this category. It was also more common among people with higher levels of education and income.[1] The study found 35% of Americans to be "low trusters," agreeing with statements that people generally cannot be trusted and will most likely take advantage of you. Those with lower incomes and less education were markedly more likely to be "low trusters." These demographic characteristics align with what I have argued throughout this book, that the particular ways in which racial minorities and lower-income individuals have been abandoned by the healthcare system and social safety net have contributed immensely to feelings of mistrust and even conspiracy.

Interestingly, the largest category, at 41% of Americans, was "medium trusters," who give relatively mixed responses to standard trust questions.[1] This suggests that there is what is sometimes referred to as a "movable middle," a large group of people who may be on the fence, between trusting and not trusting. It is critical to reach these individuals with interventions to improve trust, in part because there are so many of them, but also because there is a key opportunity to keep them from falling into an entrenched state of mistrust.

The Pew study also found that there was an obvious relationship between interpersonal trust and institutional trust: the higher someone was on the interpersonal trust scale, the more institutional trust they had, suggesting that these types of trust could be targeted together, rather than treated separately.[1] It may make sense in certain instances to focus on interpersonal trust, since more people have faith in its ability to be restored, and the interventions to address it are more obvious and more practical, including small gestures and activities to make people feel more involved and included in their local communities. Importantly, this is where healthcare also comes into the picture, with the notion that smaller, local policy changes to improve healthcare and education could also be effective at improving institutional trust.[1]

When it comes to institutional trust, it is difficult these days to discuss the concept without reference to the COVID-19 pandemic. Many studies have now examined what drove trust or mistrust during the pandemic, some of which are discussed in Chapter 4 of this book about the COVID response and about government communication processes that either helped or hindered citizens' trust in both federal and local responses. One study from 2021 by Qing Han and colleagues found surprisingly, and in contradistinction to the Pew study from 2019, that personal financial strain and employment status did not have a significant impact on overall trust in government regarding pandemic control.[2] Given the general finding from Pew and in the literature on trust that these aspects are normally associated with levels of trust, Han's finding suggests the possibility that the pandemic was a special situation in which normal correlates of institutional trust and mistrust were not necessarily at play.

Other findings from the Han study about the correlates of institutional trust during the pandemic are not too surprising. For example, higher perception of the government's level of organization in response to the pandemic, more fairness, clearer messages on coping with COVID-19, and more knowledge on COVID-19 were associated with higher levels of overall trust. Perceived knowledge and message clarity on COVID-19, fairness, and personal financial strain had direct associations with willingness to adopt recommended health behaviors. Although personal financial strain did not have a directly observable effect on trust levels, it did have an impact on willingness to adopt associated health behaviors, which suggests there may have been a level of implicit distrust for people who were suffering more financially.[2] In other words, financial strain may have impacted people's trust in the government without them necessarily being explicitly aware of it. The perceived level of the government's organization also had a direct association with prosocial behavior but not health behavior, and perceived knowledge and message clarity around COVID-19, fairness, and unemployment were directly associated with prosocial behavior.[2]

It is worth noting that the one constant in all of these measures of attitudes and behaviors is the concept of "fairness." This notion of "fairness" seems to have had an outsize effect on levels of institutional trust as well as on behaviors, both health-related and general prosocial behaviors, during the pandemic. Prosocial behaviors include things such as volunteering, donating money, and generally helping others in the community. During the pandemic, prosocial behaviors might include actions like masking, social distancing, and getting vaccinated to protect others. As discussed throughout this book, inequities have an enormous capacity to unseat trust, which can in some cases lead to poor health decision-making and belief in misinformation and even conspiracy theories. It should not necessarily surprise us that the notion of fairness was such a strong influencer in the context of the pandemic response, driving a range of attitudes and behaviors. We also know that the United States has an unusually high level of disparities in areas such as income and healthcare compared to other developed countries and that the pandemic laid these issues bare and made them even more obvious. In this context, then, it makes sense that there was such distrust and resistance to the uptake of health behaviors such as social distancing, mask wearing, and vaccination, when we put these behaviors in the context of healthcare and social systems that clearly favor some citizens over others.

This relationship between inequity and loss of trust has led some to argue that the decline in trust in the United States over the past few decades has something to do not only with increasing income inequality, but also with resentment of the display of wealth by the wealthiest 1% of society.[3–6] The idea is that distrust has grown in both government and financial institutions, because neither has intervened successfully (or even shown much of an interest in or effort to intervene).[7] Of course, there have also been many government actions and behaviors that have contributed to distrust. Abuse of power, which is closely related to corruption and scandals, has been on display at various moments across the past several decades. In addition, higher degrees of ideological conflict, which we can certainly see right now in the polarization of the political right and left, is associated with higher levels of distrust.[8,9]

The main tactic to rebuild trust in societies like the United States has been to pass laws and institute policies that are fair, transparent, applied consistently, and implemented efficiently. Periods of growth in progressive taxation in the United States and legislation to establish the welfare state represent epochs in which trust in the government was higher.[7] Some people believe, probably correctly, that it is harder to restore trust now because institutions have become more numerous, more remote, and more complex. It is also harder because distrust has increased in a broad range of institutions, including those that were not distrusted before (such as the media, the military, and higher education).[7]

There is also a newer argument that people distrust institutions because they believe they know better than the institutions. There's a certain narcissism in this, in which trust in institutions is now just an extension of partisan identity.[7] It is harder to reform because it doesn't depend on events or education—these no longer drive trust in institutions. According to this argument, the passage of new, fairer, and more transparent laws by the government will probably not be enough to restore trust. Instead, a variety of institutions in which distrust is growing need to be reformed, and some of these reforms need to be more extensive and more systemic than simply launching campaigns to display why these institutions should be trusted. Take the media, for example. Many have tried and failed to restore trust in the media. Strategies of containment of disinformation or actual litigation against the worst offenders (e.g., Alex Jones, OAN) hold promise, but they will only take out the worst offenders.[7] On a more systemic level, better funded local news would help, which would require restoring a media ecosystem that has been decimated in recent years.[10] Local news keeps people of all walks of life engaged in real news stories that connect them to their communities, and we have already shown how connection to community, as opposed to isolation, can help grow and foster trust. Giant corporations that tend to own the local news organizations that are still standing would also need to step aside, and government contribution to public media would need to be ramped up.

This response to disinformation by some of the worst offenders is still important because disinformation goes hand in hand with distrust in media (and, by extension, other institutions). It also goes hand in hand with partisan polarization and "epistemic separation," which has to do with the fact that different people have access to completely different information about the same thing. This divergence in information sources is caused by a highly partisan media environment, which has been enabled by long-term structural changes in the way the media system works in the United States. It has less to do with the situation, education, and personalities of the people consuming the information, and more to do with the fact that if you have a partisan media system, disinformation and distrust are going to grow.[11,12]

Confronting Misinformation: Theories and Interventions

It is true that combating distrust in institutions, including the healthcare system and medical professionals, is not an easy feat. There are few interventions that have actually been tested, and even fewer that most experts are particularly optimistic about. The best interventions that exist are systemic and therefore somewhat difficult to implement, including reform of the media ecosystem and improving equity in society. Local community engagement is an area that could be more amenable to change and could have a sizable impact on trust.

However, there is an important driver and consequence of distrust that may be more movable: misinformation. As discussed earlier in this chapter, the information ecosystem is an important component of people's trust in institutions and systems. When trust begins to fray, mis- and disinformation become more appealing. I will spend the second part of this chapter focusing on theories behind what drives the appeal of misinformation and what can be done to intervene to prevent its spread and people's belief in it.

What makes misinformation so appealing? One theory is simply that misinformation tends to get repeated so many times that it starts sounding like the truth. This idea, called the "illusory truth" theory, is one of the simplest explanations for the appeal and spread of misinformation. The idea here is that once something is repeated, it begins to appear plausible, and unfortunately prior knowledge does not always protect people against illusory truth. Illusory truth is also not moderated by thinking styles such as analytical versus intuitive reasoning.[13] The illusory truth effect may be bolstered by the ways in which people do and do not pay attention, especially when consuming information online. This is the heart of the "inattention theory," which suggests that people basically intend to share correct information, but the social media atmosphere prevents them from making news-sharing decisions that are consistent with the desire for accuracy.[13] At the same time, people who deliberate more and have higher numeracy skills are consistently able to discern between true and false news regardless of whether it is consonant with their political views.[13]

An opposing viewpoint suggests that inattention and illusory truth are not the drivers of misinformation. Instead, some posit that the culprit is "motivated reasoning," in which information is analyzed according to identity goals it may serve, not just according to accuracy. This theory holds that people look for information to affirm their identities, whether they be political or social identities. This means that information is distorted in order to fit our sense of self. It also means that acquiring access to the most accurate information is not the goal. According to this view, information deficits or lack of receptive capacity are not the primary drivers of susceptibility to misinformation.[13] This means that whether or not people are cognitively engaged and how much they know about the topic will make no difference in their ability to assess the accuracy of information. They will always deem the information that best confirms their identity as the most accurate. This might at least partially explain why even when high-literacy people look for health information, they have a tendency to use low-quality sites. In one study, 96% of people used low-quality sites to answer at least one question.[14]

Psychologist Stephan Lewandowsky and others have suggested that we are currently living in an information ecosystem that is a consequence of strategic extremism. In the emergence of strategic extremism, in which politicians purposely vie for the attention of those at an extreme if they will gain more votes than they will lose at the center and the other side, a precondition for success is a fractured media landscape in which information can be selectively channeled to people who are likely to support it without alienating others.[15] Long-term effects of strategic extremism may include persistence of misinformation in large segments of society when this narrowly intended set of information leaks out into the mainstream.

There is a major impediment to correcting misinformation, which has largely stumped researchers over the past decade or so. It is generally referred to as the "continued influence effect," or CIE, and refers to the phenomenon in which people continue to use incorrect information to inform their ideas and decisions, even though they have actively acknowledged a correction to misinformation. It represents one of the biggest challenges to purely fact-based approaches to misinformation, in which misinformation is corrected with updated factual information.

The continued influence effect is an important and generally pervasive phenomenon, but what causes it is more difficult to ascertain. Why would someone consciously acknowledge that information is false and then continue to utilize that false information, which they know is false, to make important decisions and inform important opinions? It seems highly irrational. Some researchers think the inclination comes in part from the way we formulate and update our so-called mental models. A mental model is a representation based on the available information and a person's knowledge about a topic, built on the principle of cause-effect relationships.[16] That is, we generally use mental models to explain and account for things that happen in our environment. If my house burns down and I discover that I left a burning cigarette in the trash, my mental model for the event of my house burning down will consist of my ideas about the cause, that I left the burning cigarette in the trash. That will be the short, but surprisingly powerful, narrative I tell myself about this event in my life.

But what happens if I suddenly get new information about this event? What if, after I have decided that the cigarette caused my house to burn down, an investigation reveals that an electrical circuit overload, probably related to outdated or worn-out electrical wiring and no fault of my own, actually caused the fire? Logic and reason would suggest that I would simply update my mental model with the new cause and throw out the old one. But there is strong evidence to suggest that this might not happen. I might instead try very hard to discount the new explanation, perhaps by faulting the investigation, looking for small uncertainties or incompetencies on the part of the people who carried it out. Or I might acknowledge the correct information but still continue to say, "I need to quit smoking because look how my negligence burned down my house." Now in this case, the result is a positive and healthy behavior change. But if we switch the topic to, say, the observation of childhood seizures after a vaccine, the resistance is not so innocuous.

Mental models are not static—they can be changed either locally when small alterations are presented, or globally when an entire model is reconstructed or a new one is created.[16] But even when someone adjusts their mental model to incorporate new information, they still might use the old misinformation to make decisions and form beliefs. The hardest mental models to change are when misinformation is part of a causal explanation in the model. Take, for example, the burning house scenario from just above. Assumptions or misinformation about the causes of the house burning down have to be overturned when new information appears on the scene. This kind of adjustment is particularly difficult for most people because the rest of the model might appear inconsistent when the misinformation is removed. Most people would prefer to keep an inaccurate but consistent mental model rather than adopt a more accurate model that is inconsistent with their general understanding of an event.[16]

Another model suggests that CIE arises from selective recall of misinformation and occurs when there is insufficient suppression of misinformation in the brain's memory centers. Misinformation might then be recalled as part of automatic memory recall processes that occur as context-free recognition of familiar information in the brain.[16] When memory is used more strategically, utilizing additional context such as source and truthfulness of information, misinformation is less likely to be brought up from memory incorrectly. This kind of operation of memory requires the utilization of sometimes significant cognitive resources. The problem is, automatic memory processes are quite common and contribute to people's decision-making more often than they should.[16]

It is important to keep the phenomenon of CIE in mind when designing and disseminating retractions of misinformation. Retractions are most likely to be successful when these factors are present: (1) warnings about subsequent exposure to misinformation—making people aware that they might encounter misinformation later and what it might look like; (2) repetition of the retraction; and (3) providing an alternative to the misinformation that fills the potential causal gap left by the retraction.[16] The most effective strategy is a combination of warning and providing an alternative to the misinformation, which is more successful than any of these items on their own.[16] Yet all of these techniques are also problematic in some way: none of them can eliminate the impact of misinformation, and sometimes the alternative is completely ineffective. Finding a credible alternative is often impossible (if it doesn't exist in the known world's body of knowledge), and warning people before they encounter misinformation can be impractical. We cannot anticipate every new piece of misinformation that may be about to drop, and even if we could, we may not have enough "foot soldiers" to get the message out to warn people before the new misinformation appears.[16] Workforce and capacity issues are a major problem in the fight against misinformation.

In the case of new misinformation, what we really want people to do is have the capacity to suspend their belief until they can verify the information (or find out it is false). It turns out that suspending belief when consuming new information is actually very unnatural for most people. It requires a high degree of attention, considerable implausibility of the message (e.g., the message really needs to reach the level of absolute absurdity to qualify for this), or high levels of distrust at the time the message is received.[15] Some scholars who study information processing have even argued that in order for a person to even process information on a basic level, they must first assume, even if for a brief period, that it is true. Otherwise, the brain power required to process the very words in the message may not be available to us.[15] In the rare cases that people are really motivated to evaluate the truth value of a message, they attend only to a few specific factors, including: (1) Is the information compatible with other things I hold true? (2) Is the information internally coherent? (3) Does the information come from a credible source? (4) Do other people believe it?[15] We could see where people might get into trouble here, especially with that last one. Internal consistency and other people's level of belief are not the best signals of the truth value of new information. It is possible and likely, especially if the misinformation is crafted by a motivated individual, that the narrative or way of communicating the information makes it seem consistent, and that many people fall for this trick, but it still doesn't make the information itself any closer to being true. And relying on what people think is a credible source may also pose some problems, as people believe anything familiar is trustworthy, so a source they read regularly may be deemed a "credible source," even if it isn't.

The source of a retraction and how the retraction is approached also matter greatly in determining whether people will incorporate the new information into their information ecosystem. There is a psychological phenomenon called "reactance," according to which people do not like retractions from an authoritative source because they feel they are being told what to do or what to think. As a result, they "react" against the retraction by holding on to misinformation.[15] In studies of mock jury situations, conviction rates tend to be higher when a judge retracts information deemed inadmissible for reasons accompanied by an extensive explanation versus situations in which information is retracted with no explanation.[15] In other words, people will hold on to the old evidence, which is now misinformation, to spite the judge who is lecturing them, but will correctly update their understanding of the situation when no one lectures them.

A few other approaches to retractions may be important to review. One inclination might be to repeat the true information until it drowns out the misinformation. It is possible that this might work in certain instances, although for whatever reason, repetition of misinformation is usually more powerful to people than repetition of corrective information, so this tactic might not be powerful enough.[15] When issuing a retraction, it may be effective to expose the motive behind the misinformation (if there is one). There is, however, a caveat to this method as well. People prefer simple information to complex information, so if a complex motive-laden explanation is provided in place of a simpler set of misinformation, people will still prefer to hold on to the misinformation rather than seriously engage with the more complex explanation of source motive.[15]

What happens when a retraction threatens someone's worldview? If the misinformation is tied to a sense of identity or is related to how someone makes sense of the world more generally, it is particularly difficult to dislodge it. However, there has been some research on the use of self-affirmation to counteract the impact of worldview-threatening retractions. This means giving people an opportunity to reflect on and affirm their identities in the process of providing the retraction. This may be as simple as asking people to write a few sentences about a time they felt really good about something because they acted according to their values before providing a retraction.[15] While this approach is certainly promising, it may not be practical outside a controlled experimental setting, especially in online interactions, when a lot of information is being shared at once and there may not be time to ensure that every single person has an opportunity to affirm themselves before being confronted with a worldview-threatening retraction.

What about crowdsourcing and letting the "crowd" correct misinformation? Surely there is some collective wisdom here, or so the thought goes. It is true that in a world where professional fact-checkers do provide correctives to misinformation, there are just not enough resources to ensure that every piece of misinformation can be corrected. This can actually lead to something called the "implied truth effect," where people start to assume that information must be accurate if it is not accompanied by a warning or a "misinformation" label.[17] In a 2018 study, Gordon Pennycook, a psychologist, and David Rand, a cognitive scientist and social psychologist, looked at the possibility of using laypeople and crowdsourcing to tag the reliability of certain web resources (not individual articles or pieces of information). They wanted to do this study because it is not at all clear that laypeople are equipped to judge the reliability of news outlets. In fact, other studies show that laypeople judge true news stories as false up to 40% of the time and judge false stories as true up to 20% of the time.[17] There is also the concern that judges of accuracy of news outlets will be motivated by partisan considerations and therefore sites that are very partisan might be judged as more accurate: the wisdom of the crowds will become the bias of the crowds. However, some of this idea has been questioned in recent research, in which it seems that misinformation belief may arise more from lack of reasoning than from motivated reasoning. This was still very much an open empirical question at the time this experiment was done.[17]

Findings from this study suggested some fact-checking success in relying on the "wisdom" of the crowd. There were a few caveats, however. Most importantly, fact-checking accuracy was not the same across partisan divides. Republicans tended to be more rigid in sticking to whatever information was most congruent with their preexisting ideas. This is consistent with the literature, which suggests that there are key systematic differences in the thinking patterns of liberal and conservatives, where conservatives show more cognitive rigidity, less tolerance for ambiguity, are more sensitive to threat, and have a greater need for order, structure, and closure.[17] Fluid thought processes that allow for rapid changing of opinion when misinformation is corrected is not thought to be a forte of the conservative way of thinking.

Combating Misinformation: The Good, the Bad, and the Ugly

I have already touched on a few methodologies thought to be effective in combating misinformation. Given the gargantuan challenges of a myriad of cognitive biases and the continued influence effect, countering misinformation is never as easy as it would seem, and it is almost never a matter of simply giving people the correct facts. While there are a variety of proposals out there about how to combat misinformation, most interventions generally fall into one of a few categories, most notably: fact-checking, priming, and inoculation. I will discuss each of these in turn.

Fact-Checking

Fact-checking is often a necessary, albeit insufficient, component of correcting and combating misinformation. What sorts of factors make a debunking message more powerful? More detailed fact-checks lead to improved quality of reasoning among participants and longer retention.[18]

Narrative corrections are more effective than non-narrative corrections in changing attitudes and behavioral intentions when the corrections are algorithmically driven, but when corrections come from members of the social media network, straight factual information, not told in story form, may be more effective.[18] Corrections that are more elaborate and engage our more rational, "System 2" thinking centers are also usually more successful.[18] As discussed earlier, debunking messages must be sufficiently detailed to allow people to build new mental models.[19] The more detailed a debunking message is, the stronger the debunking effect. The downside here, however, is that more detailed debunking messages tend to spur on a stronger continued influence effect as well.

Debunking messages are often more powerful if they somehow account for the emotions of the intended audience. In one powerful experiment, there were two conditions within the scenario that parents needed to decide whether to send their children to kindergarten during a measles outbreak knowing that some children were not vaccinated due to parents' concerns about the measles-mumps-rubella (MMR) vaccine.[20] In Condition A, there was misinformation that was corrected by the Ministry of Health but did not take into account the fears or motivations of the posting mother (who posted misinformation on the parent message board) and the other parents. Condition B included a statement that did take these fears and motivations into account and directly addressed them. Participants were then asked a series of both closed and open-ended questions about attitudes toward vaccines, how they would decide whether to send their kids to school, vaccination intentions now and in the future, and which sources of information they would trust in this situation. These questions were asked both after the misinformation was presented and then again after the Ministry of Health's response. Participants considered the information in Condition B to be considerably more trustworthy than the information in Condition A. Among hesitant parents, the reliability of the ministry's response was significantly higher in Condition B than in Condition A.[20] In short, this study found that fact-checking that is accompanied by empathic messaging is more effective, at least in the case of MMR vaccine hesitancy among concerned parents, than straight, unemotional restoration of the facts.

At the moment, fact-checking is usually completed by professional fact-checkers who spend their time scanning the Internet for misinformation and correcting large-scale false notions using clear communication of the data and evidence supporting the facts. Fact-checking is essential, but there are several problems with this approach. For one, fact-checking is incredibly time-consuming and often requires the careful work and collaboration of experts. As a result, it is not always able to be deployed that quickly, and sometimes by the time it is put forth, the misinformation has already been repeated so frequently that it is more difficult to dislodge.

Another problem is that fact-checking is really about correcting incorrect information, but sometimes misinformation is built around a kernel of truth, and that scenario can be much more difficult to fact-check.[21] In addition, fact-checking works only when there are alternative narratives to the misinformation that is being peddled. Sometimes, as has often been the case during the COVID-19 pandemic, we may know certain information is false, but we also don't have any current, true information to fill the void. The reason this was so common during COVID-19 was because the information ecosystem was constantly evolving, so at times we didn't actually have all the answers. In cases like these, we can still state why misinformation is untrue, but it is more difficult to be persuasive when we have no alternatives to fill the gap in people's mental models about a particular topic.

Finally, for all of the reasons discussed earlier in this chapter, simply correcting misinformation with up-to-date factual information often falls short of the goal. This has a lot to do with the kinds of cognitive biases most people have, the problem of the continued influence effect, and emotionally charged, identity-based issues that often resist fact-checking no matter how foolproof. So while fact-checking is often a necessary part of the equation to set the record straight, it is rarely enough to fully combat instances of misinformation.

Priming

There is some convincing evidence that "priming" people in particular ways helps combat misinformation. This means prompting people to think in a certain way before they are exposed to misinformation. For example, a study I discussed earlier that required people to complete some kind of self-affirmation by writing about a time they acted according to their values was helpful, particularly in disarming politically or ideologically motivated belief in misinformation.

Experiments that prime people to think more analytically have been shown to improve the quality of news-sharing decisions and decrease acceptance of conspiracy theories.[13] In these experiments, the hypothesis has traditionally been that people approach information in a more passive manner, not necessarily expecting that they may have to discern fact from fiction, which requires more cognitive energy than it might seem. When told to use analytical reasoning when faced with forthcoming information, people are less passive and more discerning. As a result, they are less likely to spread misinformation and probably to believe it themselves. These kinds of findings at least partially confirm the "attentional" theory of misinformation, which posits that people can be taken in by misinformation simply because they aren't paying enough attention. While priming can be an effective method, there is actually a more sophisticated version of this type of intervention, known as inoculation.

Inoculation

Inoculation may be the most effective evidence-based method of combating misinformation we have so far. Unlike fact-checking—also known as debunking, which happens after someone is exposed to misinformation— inoculation, otherwise known as prebunking, precedes exposure. The general idea is that people are exposed to a diluted version of misinformation with a warning that they are about to encounter it, which gives them a small, unappealing dose of the misinformation in a controlled environment so that if and when they face real misinformation in a more natural environment, they have already built up their arguments against it and their ability to counteract it. In this way, misinformation inoculation works very similarly to inoculation (or vaccination) against infectious diseases, by giving you a small, controlled dose of the thing itself to help you fight against it if you encounter it later in the "real" world.

Psychological inoculation treatments usually include two components: (1) a forewarning that induces a perceived threat of an impending attack on one's attitudes; and (2) exposure to a weakened micro-dose of misinformation that contains a preemptive refutation (prebunk) of the anticipated misleading arguments.[22] These components are also conceptualized as "warning" and "refutational preemption": the warning makes it visible that there are possible arguments for changing attitudes, which produces the feeling of threat. To activate the motivational processes responsible for attitude reinforcement, a person going through a process of inoculation must feel like their beliefs are in danger. Inoculation is impossible without the feeling of threat. This feeling of threat is necessary but not sufficient: preemption must also occur (e.g., exposure to arguments against one's attitude and then refutation of these arguments to strengthen one's ability to produce counterarguments to the content of future persuasion).[16]

Research has found that inoculating people against conspiratorial arguments about vaccination before exposure to a conspiracy theory effectively raised vaccination intentions.[13] In one study conducted by Jon Roozenbeek and colleagues in 2022, the experimenters inoculated participants to misinformation by focusing on common misinformation strategies, including: (1) using emotionally manipulative rhetoric to evoke emotional reactions; (2) use of incoherent or mutually exclusive arguments; (3) presenting false dichotomies or dilemmas; and (4) scapegoating individuals or groups and ad hominem attacks.[22] Subjects were presented with inoculation videos that provided a forewarning of an impending misinformation attack, then were issued a preemptive refutation of the manipulation technique used, and then finally were provided a micro-dose of misinformation. Roozenbeek and colleagues found that watching an inoculation video improved people's ability to recognize manipulation techniques and increased their confidence in their ability to do so. They also found that the videos improved subjects' ability to discern trustworthy versus untrustworthy content and improved intention around sharing (e.g., most subjects said they would not share untrustworthy information). Amazingly, this finding actually persisted 1 year later.[22] This is informative because much of the research on combating misinformation does not look at impacts beyond roughly 2 weeks.[23]

In a 2017 study, Sander van der Linden and colleagues examined the impact of an inoculation intervention on climate change misinformation. The experiment centered around consensus-building messages, which emphasized the existing scientific consensus around the fact that climate change is occurring and that it is mostly caused by human activity. Van der Linden and colleagues found that if a consensus-building message was shared followed by misinformation about climate change consensus, then the consensus message was negated completely. In other words, misinformation completely erased any potential impact of the consensus-building message.[24] On the other hand, inoculation methods were successful at maintaining the impact of consensus messages in the face of misinformation, and this actually worked across party affiliations.[24] In this study, there was no evidence of a "backfire effect," in which correcting misinformation results in a strengthening of belief in the misinformation.

Other Interventions

There are, of course, other types of interventions outside of the three types just mentioned (fact-checking, priming, and inoculation). There are a variety of other strategies that have been tested to varying degrees in the empirical literature. One area that has been tested somewhat is around narrative corrections, the idea being that telling a story as part of corrective information might be more persuasive and perhaps more "sticky" than correcting facts on its own. One study conducted by Angeline Sanalang and colleagues in 2017 consisted of two randomized-controlled trials (RCTs) to understand the potential of narrative messages to correct misinformed beliefs, attitudes, and behavioral intentions in the context of organic tobacco products. In their paper, Sanalang and colleagues explain that narratives are more salient for both attention and memory than factual corrections, and, importantly, they can immediately provide a new mental model for people where misinformation used to sit.[25] In this set of experiments, Study 1 worked in the story format, presented misinformation, and then presented a correction, which the study authors thought might work because the narrative format necessarily involves a constant updating of mental models to integrate new information. The misinformation had to do with the assertion that a supposed "natural" form of tobacco exists that is not harmful to health. They tested this against two other conditions: a narrative with no correction; and a no-exposure condition, in which no misinformation was presented. The authors also wanted to see if specific emotions improved the process of correction, so they used four different discrete emotions in the correction portion of four different conditions: fear, anger, happiness, and sadness. The study found that within-narrative corrections of misinformation were not statistically significantly better at changing attitudes than no correction or no exposure to misinformation. There was no evidence that relying on particular emotions increases the efficacy of correcting misinformation either.[25]

In Study 2, Sanalang and colleagues combined negative emotions into one condition, which was found to have a significant difference in effect on attitudes toward "natural tobacco" than the no-emotion condition. However, in all other measures, including behavioral intention, the differences were not statistically significant between simple correction (no emotion) and negative emotion correction. So the finding still holds that appeals to emotion within a narrative context did not seem to improve the response to misinformation in the most significant way: changing behaviors in response to it.[25]

Another method of fighting misinformation has to do with establishing consensus. Curious about the extent to which communicating consensus helps people hold more informed beliefs about vaccination, van der Linden and colleagues set up a study testing this relationship in 2015. In the study, subjects were randomized to one of three conditions: (1) a descriptive norm condition, in which the consensus was simply stated ("90% of scientists agree that vaccines are safe"); (2) a prescriptive norm condition, in which subjects were told that "90% of scientists agree that parents should vaccinate their children"; and (3) a control group, in which no such consensus statement was made.[26] Note that in this study, van der Linden and colleagues are not just looking at the impact of consensus statements on vaccination beliefs, but also testing the importance of the mode of delivery—descriptive (simple statement of the consensus) versus prescriptive (containing some kind of implied value judgment). The study authors then measured perceived consensus by asking what percentage of scientists agreed on safety of vaccines, perceived risk by asking how concerned people were with the risk of vaccination, and endorsement of the vaccine-autism link by asking agreement with "there is a causal link between vaccines and autism." Across the board, there was a significant effect of the consensus messaging on all dependent variables (perceived risk, acceptance of vaccine, and perception of causal link between vaccines and autism). There was furthermore no difference in results by political party or ideology.[26] The way in which the consensus statement was delivered (prescriptive or descriptive) did not seem to matter, but the existence of consensus was powerful enough to at least temporarily dissuade people from believing in vaccine misinformation. One wonders two things after reading this study: (1) how persistent these effects are, especially when people are faced with new misinformation; and (2) whether these findings would hold up today, when beliefs about vaccines and health-related matters in general have become more partisan and vitriolic.

There is also an open question about whether the source of the correction to misinformation matters and to what extent. In a creative study of 700 subjects, Toni van der Meer and Yan Jin measured several different scenarios, namely the impacts of corrective information type (factual elaboration versus simple rebuttal) and source type (news media versus government versus peer).[27] The control group received misinformation but no correction. The situation in the study was a hypothetical infectious disease outbreak. All respondents were exposed to misinformation that the virus was not a severe threat. In the simple rebuttal condition, subjects were exposed to bullet points laying out the fact that the virus is a severe threat. In the factual elaboration condition, they were given reasons why it was a severe threat. Respondents were exposed to these different types of corrective information, in combination with different types of sources, including media, government, and peer. After these exposures, a questionnaire appeared measuring emotions, sense of crisis severity, and the likelihood of taking preventive actions. Participants reported feeling more hope and less anxiety, confusion, and fear when they were exposed only to the misinformation and not also to the corrective information. Participants were not more likely to take preventive actions in response to the outbreak when they saw corrective information in addition to misinformation. Those exposed to simple rebuttal felt less anxiety and fear than those exposed to factual elaboration. Participants exposed to factual elaboration would take more preventive action than those exposed to simple rebuttal. People who received information from news media and the government perceived a greater degree of crisis severity than those who received information from a peer. Participants felt more anxiety when exposed to government and news media information versus peers. No differences were found according to source for behavioral intentions. Interestingly, news media and government did evoke a response suggesting people should take the threat seriously. On the other hand, the greater amount of fear and anxiety evoked by government sources could ultimately work against quelling misinformation because strong emotions, especially anxiety, are often associated with susceptibility to believing misinformation and an inability to give it up. It is hard to know whether behavioral intentions would translate into actual behaviors, and this is a major shortcoming of most existing research on misinformation interventions. Nonetheless, it is worth noting that none of the source types makes a difference in what people say they intend to do, suggesting that there may not be much of an advantage of a government or media source delivering corrective information versus a layperson or "peer" population. This is true in other studies too, where people lean on a sense of how much they trust someone versus their expertise, which sometimes seems to be beside the point.[28–32]

In 2020, Dominik Stecula and colleagues published a paper based on a 2019 representative sample of the American population. Granted, this was before the pandemic and the COVID-19 vaccine, which has likely changed attitudes and behaviors surrounding vaccination more generally, but some of the findings are still relevant. For example, the survey found that those who professed low trust in medical experts were more likely to believe vaccine misinformation, and this was true across demographic groups.[33] This is not necessarily an immediately obvious finding; that is, we would not necessarily expect that those who mistrust healthcare providers would automatically believe vaccine misinformation. One could argue, for example, that people with low levels of trust could potentially be more discerning and more invested in carefully examining health information and therefore might be more immune to misinformation. Instead, it does seem to be the case that these factors (low trust and belief in misinformation) coincide. While we lack great studies showing us why these two factors so frequently appear together, one possibility is that misinformation is deliberately constructed to appeal to people with preexisting low levels of trust so that the content of the misinformation conforms to their worldview that the healthcare system and U.S. healthcare authorities are not to be trusted.

Thankfully, some studies do find that even people with low levels of trust in the healthcare system still trust their own doctors and will take advice from them, as discussed more extensively in Chapter 1. And as Stecula and colleagues note, one intervention—motivational interviewing—works quite well in these doctor-patient settings (if doctors can find the time).[33] But the relationship between negative trust and misinformation is very strong. Negative trust is a stronger predictor of belief in misinformation than even some of the most oft-cited influences, including education, income, age, religiosity, and conservative news consumption.[33] Stecula and colleagues also noted the persistence of misinformed beliefs: even in cases in which people had a relatively low volume of misinformed beliefs, these beliefs persisted even 5 months later, after extensive CDC campaigning to combat misperceptions.

There are several very promising interventions to counteract misinformation. Some of the most successful to date include inoculation, priming, and attendance to values and goals. What is missing from all of the studied approaches to misinformation is a focus on the underlying mistrust. Mistrust and misinformation go hand in hand, and one can easily goad the other. I am certain that Stecula and colleagues would agree that one of the major issues with the style of campaigning in which CDC and other health agencies engage is that it does not address the underlying issue of mistrust, which is the foundation on which misinformed beliefs are born and grow. And it is because of this critically important foundation, one that is so hard to understand, measure, and respond to, that I have spent several hundred pages now exploring its roots and attempting to understand its consequences.

Just for Fun: What Does Trust-Building Look Like in Other Countries?

As you probably have noticed by now, this book is very U.S.-focused, and that is intentional, because my research focuses on the U.S. context. However, a good friend and collaborator of mine, who is also a sociologist, immediately asked, when reading parts of this book: Can you make any comparisons to different countries? While I initially experienced some psychological resistance and blamed his sociologist bias for suggesting such a cross-country comparison, I quickly realized that this was in fact a very good idea. So here, I provide a few references to how things look in Norway, Finland, and South Korea when it comes to trust and provide some concluding thoughts on where this leaves us in the United States.

Let's start with Norway. This country has a bit of pride of place in this book because, one of my most telling interviews was with a family member of someone who lived in Montana, moved to Norway, and came back to Montana. Of course, while she was in Norway she developed positive feelings about healthcare and the healthcare system, in large part because there is universal healthcare in Norway and she was suddenly able to access medical professionals. When she returned to Montana and her access was taken away, she reverted to a very high level of distrust of modern medicine and the healthcare system. This was the first clue I received for the idea that lack of healthcare access spurs on distrust. Aside from universal healthcare, Norwegians enjoy relatively high levels of trust in their government more generally. An OECD report found that a robust welfare system that offers high-quality services in Norway contributes to lower levels of inequality, which tends to be an important determiner of institutional trust in any country.[34] During the pandemic, 68% of people expressed satisfaction with control measures and 69% expressed confidence in information from the government, which is basically unheard of in the United States.[34] In addition, high rates of political participation and feelings of community belongingness contribute to national-level institutional trust, and both of these factors are relatively high in Norway.[34] The case study includes an interesting excursus on the connection between interpersonal (or social) trust and institutional trust:

> Trust in other people is comparatively high (7.25 on average). Trust in others is a crucial measuring stick of social capital. High levels of social trust indicate that citizens are positive about the moral standards in their country. It is a clear signal that citizens feel that they are part of a broader societal network. In societies where trust is widespread, all sorts of monitoring and security costs are reduced, and citizens are more likely to express solidarity towards one another. Hence, when citizens feel that they can trust most other people in their country, including strangers, migrants, people with a different economic background, etc., societies usually tend to function better, because co-operation is facilitated. . . . An empirical study with data from World Value Survey (WVS) finds a strong correlation between social (interpersonal) and political trust. According to the authors, trust in governmental institutions is shaped through social relationships and in this way, these relations also have an impact on institutional performance.[34]

In other words, high levels of trust in other individuals and a general feeling that people are honest and morally upright is not unrelated to the extent to which people trust their government institutions. These concepts are usually on a continuum in people's minds, so low levels of interpersonal and social trust can affect the extent of institutional trust in any given country.

In nearby Finland, levels of trust in the government and other institutions are similarly high. In November 2020, at the height of the pandemic, 86% of the population considered information shared by political leaders to be reliable.[35] Of course, it is important to understand that even with such high overall trust rates, there are still pockets of the population where distrust is a problem, especially among rural residents, lower-income households, and people who are less educated.[35] Nonetheless, the overall levels are still much higher than what we see here in the United States. One thing that has helped Finland maintain these high levels of trust, even during the pandemic, is that the government tends to do a good job of responding to uncertainty.[35] In general, people have the perception that the government plans ahead, and they feel that the extent of uncertainty in their environments is not overwhelmingly high.[35]

A good counterpart to these two Scandinavian examples comes from South Korea. South Korea has experienced considerable growth in wealth over the past 50 years and has a strong fiscal profile by OECD standards.[36] The trust profile in South Korea, however, is lower than one might expect given its fiscal stance. Institutional trust, particularly in the government, is still quite low.[36] Much of this distrust is likely related to the still vast inequalities that exist in South Korean society, and this finding also gives us a clue into what might be going on with trust in the United States as well. There is a pervasive feeling in South Korea that even with overall rapid financial growth over the past 50 years, that growth has been very uneven, with certain vulnerable portions of the population, including women and the elderly, largely being left behind and treated differently in key areas, including education and employment.[36] This is also a common story in the United States, where inequalities are quite sharp and visible, especially by race and income. In some ways, the high-quality healthcare we *do* have in the United States makes matters worse, since this level of care is often available only to a select few who can afford it or who have jobs at large, wealthy organizations that can afford to buy high-quality insurance coverage.

There is one more non-U.S. example to ponder, this one having to do with the regulatory environment. The European Union has been especially aggressive of late in trying to regulate the online, social media arena to inhibit the spread and influence of misinformation, which, as I have discussed throughout this chapter, is both a contributor to and a symptom of mistrust. The Digital Services Act requires that social media companies show active evidence of work they are doing to counteract misinformation on their platforms. Noncompliance with this and other provisions of the Act, which include an array of measures to reduce the spread of misinformation, can lead to up to 6% of global turnover (which is usually hundreds of millions of dollars) and ultimately to a platform being altogether banned in the European Union.[37] We need stronger measures like this in the United States, too.

These measures of overall trust in institutions and one another are important because, as I have argued, healthcare and attitudes toward it are very often at the center of both the foundation of democracy and people's overall level of trust in those who run their society. Medical mistrust is both like a virus and like a symptom—it grows and spreads its own offspring (belief in misinformation, conspiratorial thinking, and unhealthy behaviors), but it is also a symbol of a larger level of societal decay that pervades an array of other political and social institutions outside the healthcare system. In the Conclusion, I will attempt to summarize what we have learned and reflect on the very grave consequences of a society in which medical mistrust runs rampant.

Conclusion

Where Do We Go From Here?

On February 3, 2023, a privately owned train on a privately owned railway derailed and released hazardous chemicals into the air in East Palestine, Ohio. While the Environmental Protection Agency (EPA) proclaimed that the pollution was not significant enough to cause long-term health damage, many people in East Palestine felt understandably frustrated. The right-wing media immediately came up with a conspiracy theory that the train's derailment was ordered by the Biden administration on purpose to damage the lives of specifically poor White people in an old steel mill town. It feels as though every event in the United States is inevitably shrouded in a dark cloud of distrust and conspiracy theories, and sometimes that smog is so thick and so opaque that we feel absolutely lost in looking for a clear path forward.

After the previous chapters that so thoroughly examine what's wrong with our healthcare and public health systems and how these issues bespeak larger problems with our democracy, I want to leave you on a more positive note. While research into solutions to the problems of misinformation and faulty information ecosystems, the nature of our healthcare system, and restoring trust and a functioning democracy is far from decisive, there are some actions we can take to improve the situation.

First, I want to expand upon the examination of misinformation in the previous chapter. Over the years, I have found it increasingly important not only to discuss misinformation and disinformation as phenomena unto themselves, but also to look at the consumption of information in terms of "information environments." Rather than examining specific pieces of misinformation circulating in a community or an online environment, it is instead imperative that we understand the entire information ecosystem around a person or a community of people. Where do they get their information? Is this information sparse or under threat in some way? Do they gather information from multiple sources, and are multiple sources even available to them? Do they have access to verified, scientific sources of information, or only secondhand information circulating about scientific topics within a given bounded community setting? Over time, it has become increasingly clear that there are significant health equity implications of the type of information ecosystem in which a person or a community of people operate. Low-income, racial minority communities in the United States tend to have poorer information ecosystems and impoverished access to high-quality information compared to high-income, predominantly White communities. For this reason, it has become increasingly appropriate to view information environments as a social determinant of health.

It is a natural human inclination to seek out information. Human beings operate under an "information imperative," meaning that for the most part we are constantly seeking information and ways to utilize it.[1] In some ways, hunting for information is our modern version of hunting for food. A healthy information ecosystem can literally make the difference between life and death, as we have all too painfully seen during the COVID-19 pandemic.

What happens when the information ecosystem begins to get polluted? And how does this even happen in the first place? While it's unclear exactly what has happened to the information environment in the United States (and many other places in the world), there are some convincing theories. Over time, news sources in the United States have become narrower and less "fecund."[1] A "fecund" news source allows for information in more abundant context, so that people can use it to make decisions, can distinguish between patterns and one-off events, can anticipate future developments, and can thoughtfully use background information.[1] The consolidation of media sources over the past several decades has played a role in reducing fecundity and increasing polarization.[1] These new consolidated news sources tend not to represent a diversity of viewpoints and are more likely to be swayed by political and corporate pressures.[1] In short, they do not give readers the tools to consider complex topics from multiple angles, to analyze the information freely and form their own opinions, or to understand that there may be more than one way of looking at matters. This disempowers people and erodes their self-efficacy, or their belief that they can fend for themselves in the midst of complex, demanding information. In the end, many of these sources look more like propaganda than news.

The consolidation of media sources is thus one major factor in the increasingly unwell information environment in which we find ourselves at present. Then there is social media. It's always difficult to know how much to blame social media directly for any social phenomenon. That's because everyone is on it, which makes it hard to study a control group of people who have no access to or interaction with social media whatsoever. We do know, however, that the concept of the "information cascade," which allows only a few people to amplify their ideas with incredible reach and efficiency, is something that is almost certainly made much worse by social media.[2] Because of the way social media companies design their algorithms, an "influencer" or even a regular person can have wide reach across individuals who share pre-existing beliefs, thus having a rapid ability to affect behaviors in large numbers of people. This kind of rapid thought- and behavior-change mechanism involving thousands or even millions of people nearly instantly is not generally possible without social media.

This kind of dysfunction within the information environment probably requires an intervention on the level of the government, and most likely the federal government in most cases. In a 2017 study, Pew found that people who believe that the information environment will not improve much in the next 10 years also believe that powerful corporate and government forces have an important role to play in attempting to fix the problem.[3] In this same study, interestingly, many Americans readily perceived the information ecosystem problem as an equity problem.[3] Equity problems usually require government intervention—they are not something that can generally be resolved with intervention by the private sector alone. Many Americans also recognize that the emphasis on free speech in this country is a hindrance to appropriate regulation of social media sources that are in many ways infecting the information environment.[3] By way of solution, many Americans also shared that they believed in bolstering public press sources and independent journalism, as well as a focus on media literacy in all levels of education.[3]

There's also a growing consensus, on both sides of the political aisle, that social media companies need to be more extensively regulated by the federal government. Some argue that these companies need to be held accountable for content that is posted on their sites, which is not always a popular opinion.[4] This can also be difficult to achieve in practical terms because, again, of our country's understandable focus on not hindering free speech. At the very least, the government should have a better plan for how to communicate and monitor social media in times of crisis. For example, at the beginning of the COVID-19 pandemic there was intelligence from the European Union saying that Russia was trying to blame COVID-19 on biological warfare from Western countries and through this trying to reduce people's trust in the healthcare system. As we know, in moments of crisis when people are already anxious, they are more likely to believe misinformation.[5,6] The government should have had a plan for preempting and debunking this kind of disinformation. In a crisis like COVID, governments need to communicate everything promptly, even if information is not "finalized," because this is when disinformation starts to bubble up.[7] Other countries around the world have begun to set up governmental task forces to deal with mis- and disinformation. Italy has a multi-stakeholder task force as part of the government that focuses on mis- and disinformation.[7] Some countries (including Korea and Canada) are using open government portals to encourage participation by members of the general public in dissemination of information about health-related topics. This has to be done well so as not to allow for publication of misinformation coming from the government, but the participatory angle is what's important here.[7] Spain is engaged in widespread prebunking efforts—they share information about COVID alongside "possible misinformation or hoaxes" people might hear later on.[7] Colombia has set up a Public Communication of Science and Public Outreach Strategy to focus on a communication strategy especially around crises like COVID and times when quick communication is needed.[7] While some of these initiatives may fail and all of them need careful evaluation efforts, they are all reasonable actions to take and well worth it. The United States should follow in the footsteps of these other countries around the world that are taking coordinated action against the scourge of mis- and disinformation.

Remedying our Broken Healthcare System

As mentioned in the previous chapter, one of the people I interviewed while writing this book spoke eloquently about his aunt, who mistrusted healthcare and medicine while living in the United States with no health insurance and who changed her attitudes almost as soon as she moved to Norway, where healthcare was free. Upon returning to the United States, old attitudes about the crooked nature of the medical and healthcare systems came right back. I heard many similar stories (although none quite so stark) as I interviewed dozens of people about close friends and family members who have high levels of mistrust in medicine, public health, and the healthcare system.

The change in my interviewee's aunt's attitudes about health and medicine and the move from the United States to Norway and back again is probably not a coincidence. Instead, as I have argued throughout this book, healthcare access is a key determinant of trust in the health and public health systems. Our country's ability to fight off a novel pandemic or respond to any other type of health emergency is therefore in many ways dependent on how well our healthcare system covers the country's citizens. At any given time, about 20% of Americans are being actively pursued by collection agencies for healthcare debts.[8] In a typical year, a nonprofit hospital may sue around 20,000 people for payment of overdue medical bills.[9] Until the mid-1980s, hospitals could charge Medicare whatever price they wanted, but subsequently prices were capped. As a result, hospitals pushed costs onto those who were not insured or had slim coverage and started hiring MBAs to make hospitals more of a business.[8] With millions of people still completely uninsured and many more underinsured (although the CDC did report an 18% drop in the uninsured rate during the pandemic), and with healthcare expenses being one of the most common cause of bankruptcy in this country, it is fairly safe to say that access to healthcare in the United States is outrageously bad.[10-12] And it comes as no surprise that access to healthcare in a country like Norway is infinitely better. At one point, I interviewed someone from Japan who had suffered from a debilitating chronic illness her whole life. She had some level of questioning of medical professionals because she felt it took too long to treat her condition properly, which is something we hear from many who suffer from chronic illness in the United States and elsewhere. And yet, when I asked her about her access to care and global trust of medicine and healthcare, she was much more measured than her counterparts in the United States. She actively expressed a feeling of having been well taken care of and covered by her government's healthcare system and felt no broader suspicion as a result.

If we are to manage the problem of medical mistrust in this country, it is going to take more than interventions on the individual level to convince people of the importance of positive health behaviors and listening to one's medical provider. The true problem at the heart of this phenomenon is our country's broken healthcare system and, more specifically, the fact that so many people simply have no or poor access to basic healthcare. Without addressing these structural issues, individual interventions will only get us so far.

While it may be difficult to come up with a solution that satisfies both sides of the political aisle, there is at least widespread bipartisan agreement that the healthcare system needs massive reforms. In a 2020 survey, 92% of Republicans said the healthcare system needs major reforms, with Democrats and Republicans largely agreeing overall.[13] COVID revealed the problem with tying health insurance to employers and the major inadequacies of our social safety net, including the general lack of sick time and days off to care for someone who is ill.[14] The United States is a global outlier in tying health insurance to employment, which mostly came about as an accident of history, as employers offered fringe benefits to employees after World War II in a tough labor market in order to attract workers. Glaring deficits have been highlighted by the COVID-19 crisis, including problems with health insurance, sick leave, and unemployment benefits.[14] Half of all Americans, including both Democrats and Republicans, agree that they would like to buy a new federal health insurance plan that people can pay for on a sliding scale.[13] The problem is when it comes to discussing who should pay for such a plan, Democrats and Republicans predictably disagree.[13]

Fixing the American healthcare system is decidedly political (whether or not it should be) and certainly beyond the scope of this book. However, in the interest of providing a full picture of the problem of medical mistrust and some of its possible solutions, I would be remiss not to mention some of the prevailing theories on what might actually help. The "how" of some of these proposed solutions is less clear, especially in a highly partisan political environment.

One thing that has often been commented on is the fact that prevention is simply not funded in the United States.[15] CDC funding has been flat-lined for years, and there has been virtually no investment in data infrastructure for public health specifically, even though there has been considerable investment in medical data.[16] This means that even if we wanted to start investing more in public health, we might not even know where to start given the lack of data on effective interventions to improve the public's health and well-being and to prevent serious health issues at a population level. CDC funding was even being threatened and cut during the pandemic, which suggests a serious lack of overall cultural valuing of the power of prevention. Investing in data infrastructure that focuses on prevention is one obvious way forward here; knowing how to deal with cultural devaluation of prevention measures is a more difficult problem to solve.

Much of the discussion about fixing our country's healthcare crisis has focused on price transparency. At the moment, patients know little to nothing about how much different medical services will cost, and, so the theory goes, there is an information asymmetry that can result in a massive overuse of unnecessary care. This is a reasonable theory—perhaps if people knew more about what different medical options actually cost, they would make more calculated decisions about which treatments to pursue and therefore the total cost of healthcare in this country would decline. And yet, the limited number of experiments that have focused on price transparency have suggested that this may not be the solution to high healthcare costs that many people think it is.[17] In many cases, even when prices are available, patients fail to utilize this information, in part because they still need or rely on referrals from their doctor, they may not fully understand what is best for their medical condition, and they may not be equipped to assess quality differences among providers.[18]

Other countries, mostly in the European Union, have attempted to control healthcare costs and deal with access and inequity issues usually by some combination of controlling prices and offering universal healthcare. As Zeke Emanuel has aptly pointed out, universal health coverage is still a relatively new idea, and no country, not even European countries with much better healthcare systems than ours, has fully figured it out yet.[14] Still, simply establishing universal healthcare does improve access issues considerably. On the price front, some countries have set up separate bodies to determine costs to create a separation between cost determination and the political calculation of negotiating prices. Characteristics of these types of bodies are political independence, formal systems of communication with stakeholders, and freedom from conflicts of interest.[7] Unilateral prices set by a central government body are the best option, something we mostly do not do in the United States. Individual negotiations among sellers and buyers encourages price discrimination and growth of healthcare costs.[7] The OECD also recommends investment in data infrastructure so that detailed information about costs and quality can be recorded and analyzed.[7] In the United States, we do this spottily at best.

There are other steps that could be taken short of an overhaul of the entire healthcare system. Perhaps children could be covered on insurance plans at no additional cost, for example.[14] The United States is the only country that puts so much pressure on the family to pay for children's healthcare.[14] Even in situations with private healthcare, perhaps the government could pay for children's healthcare. Most children are healthy and do not require enormous sums of money in healthcare bills. While having the government set prices for certain types of healthcare expenditures can result in inequities, capping prices has been shown to be relatively useful and efficient.[17] Community health centers could be expanded, especially as these venues have gained bipartisan support over the years.[19] Federal funding for Federally Qualified Health Centers (FQHCs), which provide comprehensive health services usually in underserved areas, also needs to be expanded.[19] Financing school-based clinics is another avenue to provide more free healthcare especially to children.[19]

Why does access to healthcare matter so much in a discussion of trust and conspiracy theories? My suspicion that the direction of causality flows from low access to mistrust and susceptibility to conspiracy theories and misinformation is quite clear. We know, for example, that having health insurance coverage has been significantly associated with lower odds of believing misinformation about COVID-19.[20] In one study, having health insurance was the only significant predictor of plans to vaccinate a child against flu and was a major predictor of plans to vaccinate a child against COVID-19.[21] We also know that trust in the healthcare system affects very real decisions that could change the course of a person's health and life. One study on vaccination to prevent human papillomavirus (HPV), which also protects against cervical cancer and certain types of nasopharyngeal cancer, found that there were high levels of awareness in the general population about the connection between HPV and cancer and the fact that the HPV vaccine is an anti-cancer vaccine. Nonetheless, a strong reluctance to vaccinate teens against HPV came from a general distrust of the healthcare system.[22] In other words, even when people understand that a preventive measure might prevent cancer, one of the worst possible outcomes that any parent can imagine for their child, they still did not want to opt for vaccination due to a general unease with the healthcare system.

We also know that excessive spending on healthcare can cause lower wages throughout the population and less spending on other government services, including important social services that form the basis of our social safety net, such as unemployment and housing benefits.[23] In other words, when healthcare spending gets out of control, everyone is affected, but especially people who really need the government to operate a functional social safety net. This leads to further inequities in our society, which, as discussed throughout this book, can exacerbate polarized political tensions and ultimately lead some people down a path to extreme views.

There is no easy fix to our healthcare woes in this country. The issue is both extremely complex and extremely political. But if we continue to do nothing and make very little of an effort to improve the situation, I am confident that more and more people will continue to fall down the well of conspiracy theories and misinformation and our health as a population will continue to erode at an alarming rate. The suggestions here are a mere beginning— but we have to start somewhere. Importantly, a good first step is to understand the connection between the healthcare system's dysfunction and the feelings of distrust many people have in health and medicine. This is a major part of the argument of this book, and I hope I have succeeded in making clear that these phenomena are intimately interconnected. The problem of medical mistrust and conspiracy theories in this country will not be resolved unless structural issues around the healthcare system, including poor access to healthcare and systemic racism in medicine and healthcare, are at least somewhat addressed.

Restoring Trust

Addressing systemic healthcare issues is part of the equation of increasing trust in healthcare and medicine, but it is probably not the whole picture. In wrapping up this gargantuan and complex topic of "trust," it is well worth our while to review some of the basic tenets of what human trust is, how it is formed and how it is broken, and, finally, what are some ways it can be restored.

At the most basic level, we might ask ourselves: Is trust uniquely human? We know that chimpanzees, some of our closest neighbors, experience a form of preferential "interpersonal trust," in that they come to trust their friends more than their non-friends.[24] Chimpanzees also show signs of spontaneous trust and the ability to modify their trust over time based on the trustworthiness of the other actor.[25] They also engage in a kind of "testing the waters" behavior in which they give other chimpanzees increasingly complex tasks to see if they can be trusted with independent projects.[26] Scholars who study chimpanzees have also identified the "cooperative leap of faith," in which a chimpanzee gives another chimpanzee an extremely important task as a test, such as watching one's baby.[26] Human beings engage in similar forms of "trust-testing" experiments, testing others to see if they are worthy of our full trust and faith. Of course, there is also a degree of random, immediate judgment that occurs in both animals, that may lead us to decide we trust or do not trust someone almost instantaneously. This form of trust formation is harder to study and understand but makes up a good proportion of the trust judgments we make on a regular basis.

While chimpanzees are almost always surrounded by other animals they know, human beings spend much of the time in the company of strangers. Forming trust emotions toward a complete stranger is a uniquely human phenomenon that basically does not exist in the animal kingdom.[26] In the end, trust is about believing that someone is going to behave in a predictable pattern, in accordance with how you think they are going (and perhaps expect them) to behave.[27] In human beings and probably in chimpanzees as well, this trust and expectation are formed on the basis of observation of previous behavior.[26] In arguably simpler beings, such as fish and guppies, animals in the species have so much genetic similarity that they all behave in the same fashion and no one has to observe individual behaviors to know whether or not to trust a single individual member of the species.[26] In the wild, being an untrustworthy individual can be downright dangerous: young coyotes who invite others to play and then play roughly or deceive them in some other way tend to be ostracized, leave their pack, and go off on their own, where they usually suffer higher mortality.[26] Trust doesn't need a language or a society to exist and be important, but in most species, being a trustworthy individual is desirable and sometimes key to survival. Human beings also strive to be trusted, as it increases the ability to join groups, and we know that joining groups is adaptive to human survival and the ability to thrive. There are enormous benefits of trust on both the interpersonal and the societal levels. Trusting relationships bolster health and mental health, and countries that enjoy higher levels of interpersonal trust tend to flourish more economically.[28,29]

Given the importance of trust to society and survival, we might think the trust judgment is a long, drawn-out process, associated with elevated cognition and effort. On the contrary, trust judgments are often made in split seconds. The estimate is that it takes most humans one-tenth of a second to decide whether or not they trust someone, usually based on a broad judgment about the features of a person's face.[30] Perhaps not surprisingly, there is a tendency to overgeneralize trust judgments and, on the flip side, to discount entire groups of people based on snap trust judgments about a single individual who might belong to that group.[31] In my previous book *Denying to the Grave: Why We Ignore the Science That Will Save Us*, I spent a great deal of time discussing psychological heuristics or shortcuts that result in the misjudgment of complex scientific information. Here too we see a socially driven heuristic at play in which a judgment that should take multiple encounters, observation, and some deep thought occurs almost automatically, based on mostly peripheral cues that may or may not be meaningful. Once again, our favorite activity—taking shortcuts—is a key component of this human process.

What happens when trust erodes on the societal or country level, not just on the interpersonal level? The two are in fact intertwined. Low community and governmental trust tend to go hand in hand, and they negatively reinforce each other.[32] In a country such as Brazil, in which low trust in the political and social systems is present in about 70% of the population, we also see that about 63% of the population reports not trusting other people in their communities.[32] While it is possible to see one type of trust flourishing while the other recedes, it is more often the case that the two mirror each other. This means that any intervention we choose to deal with eroding trust on the societal level should also repair trust on the interpersonal, community level as well.

One area that certainly deserves our attention is the information environment. There is a gross miscalculation people make when they talk to each other: that everyone has access to the same information. As discussed elsewhere in this book, there are serious inequities in the extent to which individual citizens and communities are able to access high-quality, accurate information about a variety of topics, including health and medical information, information about the environment, political information, and many other topics.[33–35] The assumption that others have access to all the same information you do can cause communications that come off as condescending and can ultimately cause a loss in trust. I believe this is much of what is behind the loss of people's trust in the CDC during the pandemic.

Interventions on the Small Scale Could Show Promise

I will admit that there were times in the midst of writing this book when I did feel somewhat helpless (and hopeless). I was regularly talking to people who had lost most or all of their faith in medicine and the healthcare system, some of whom did have terrible stories about ways that their pain was dismissed, ways that they were neglected in the course of care, or ways that they just couldn't get the care they needed, due to expenses, where they lived, or other reasons related to access. But many of the conversations I had with family members of those who had lost their faith in the healthcare system helped me emerge from this feeling that all was lost. In these conversations, I happened to stumble upon a simple fact: interventions conducted by family members to increase the trust in and reduce belief in conspiracy theories around health and medicine have a good chance at being effective. Here's a little bit about what I heard:

- In many cases, people could point to interventions or interactions that worked, but they often couldn't tell me why. One man whose father was so distrustful of the healthcare system that he outright refused to go on a statin after having a heart attack, who spent all his time searching for and watching fringe news sources, and who believed that COVID was a government conspiracy to pave the path to a one-world government, told me that his father's mother (his grandmother) had an amazing and almost unbelievable capacity to "talk sense" into her son. My interviewee was not always present for these conversations, but he watched as his grandmother gently expressed her concerns and asked her son empathic questions to get a better feeling for what he was so afraid of. This person said with absolute certainty that his father would be much worse off, maybe even not alive, if it were not for his grandmother and these gentle conversations and nudges to keep him looking after his health, at least on the most basic level.
- Even when interviewees thought they were making somewhat of a difference, they always told me they wished they had more tools at their disposal. One woman dealt with a situation with her mother that was absolutely tragic, with her mother eventually dying prematurely most likely because she refused to see a doctor for severe abdominal pain. Her mother also stopped leaving the house in her later years, and it seemed to her daughter like she was almost part of a cult that spread conspiracy theories about health and medicine on social media. Despite her mother's extreme beliefs and her eventual tragic death, this woman told me that she did think she had some productive conversations with her mother over the years. She would affirm things that she thought might be helping her mother, like acupuncture or physical therapy, while gently questioning things that seemed less helpful and more on the fringes of the evidence around health-promoting behaviors. I could tell that these conversations had been extremely difficult for her, and she was incredibly courageous in taking them on. She told me she really wished she had more tools to be able

to have these conversations even more effectively—perhaps that could have even prevented her mother's death.

- Some individuals tried to empower their family members and impart skills to them that would give them the self-efficacy to evaluate evidence for themselves and feel effective and accomplished in this venture. As I've argued in other places in this book, self-efficacy is an extremely important part of the equation in counteracting misinformation and conspiracy theories. Self-efficacy is so important in part because many people believe that they don't have the capacity to evaluate scientific evidence and come to rely too heavily on questionable ideas due to a sense that they always need extensive guidance and people telling them essentially "what to think." One woman whose parents are immigrants from Pakistan who held a lot of distrustful views of medicine and health shared that she regularly tries to teach her parents how to evaluate evidence, and that in many cases, this works. Sometimes they would revert back to old beliefs after a few days, but this cycling suggests that there are opportunities for intervention. Distrust in healthcare and conspiracy theory belief do not actually have to be constant, and in many cases they probably are not. Instead, people wax and wane—sometimes their beliefs are stronger and sometimes they are weaker. When someone who observes them frequently, like a family member, notices this waning, that is a perfect time to intervene.

- Persistence is often key, and family members are well situated to repeatedly nudge someone toward a particular health behavior. When the COVID pandemic started and talk arose about a new vaccine, one of my interviewees was very concerned about her father, who lived in a small town that had a history of anti-vaccine and anti-science sentiment. Her father was always terrified of most foods, to the point where she felt he had developed an eating disorder because of his obsession with "clean," pesticide-free, organic food. He refused to eat at restaurants and he thought salad bars were sprayed with chemicals. When the vaccines came out for COVID-19, she was particularly worried that her father wouldn't get the shot, so she started early and often, nudging and reminding him to get the shot. Eventually, he did get it, and she attributes a lot of this success to her persistence.

- Some interviewees tried a tactic that has a good evidence base in the literature, around asking people to explain their beliefs in more detail. As discussed above, one person told me stories about his aunt, who had grown up in rural Montana and lived a relatively isolated life. She subscribed to some relatively extreme conspiracy theories, including the idea that there's a microchip in the COVID vaccines, that COVID was invented to cover up a world plot surrounding 5G technology, and even that jet lines from a plane are really chemicals from the government put into the air to harm and control the population. She also believes that viruses don't exist, especially AIDS. Her isolation proved especially harmful during the pandemic, when she would disconnect her power for 23 hours a day and refuse to use her phone because of a conspiracy theory involving the electrical grid. While my interviewee opined that his aunt's views were really like a religion and potentially not movable, he did share that he occasionally has some success by asking her to explain her ideas more fully. For example, he would ask her, "if AIDS doesn't exist, then why did all those people die?" She would in those moments hesitate. There is a vast literature that suggests that people think they know more than they actually do.[36] For example, most people claim to know how a zipper works, but when you actually ask them to explain it, they falter. In the case of conspiracy theories and misinformation, this factor might be used to open up space in a conversation where we can get a person to question their beliefs by helping them realize that they don't fully understand them. In some cases, this might not work very well if someone is too radicalized, but in many cases, knowing how to open up the conversation is half the battle and can lead to a more rational discussion.

This is only a smattering of examples of the ways that the people I spoke to tried to intervene with their family members. Everyone I spoke to expressed a great deal of distress and concern for their loved ones, and most were unwilling to give up on them and would be willing to try an array of strategies to help change their viewpoints. There is a lot more we can do with this information. We can first of all collect many more examples of these kinds of "private" interventions, and we can utilize them to craft robust interventions that can actually be tested. I do believe that some of our best ideas might come from people who are struggling with conspiratorial beliefs every day (or at least very frequently), who are naturally trying an array of potentially successful strategies. In these small interventions, we might very well have the seeds for something extremely effective and game-changing when it comes to moving people with high levels of distrust and conspiratorial beliefs that are in many cases putting their health at serious risk.

Restoring Democracy

Throughout this book, I have made the argument that the dire problems with our healthcare system and the loss of trust in it are related to the various ways in which our democracy is failing. Most obviously, the response to the COVID pandemic was a grand display of the broken trust between the American people and the public health and political systems and the conspiracy theories and extremist views that this broken trust have caused. In a less obvious fashion, the slow erosion of trust in the healthcare system and the failure of the health and social safety net in this country have created an atmosphere of despair and disillusionment that have crafted the perfect environment for extremist political ideas to arise. Angus Deaton and Anne Case have already argued eloquently that the out-of-control costs of the healthcare system have had downstream effects on the economy that have led to an epidemic of despair. In this book, I have argued further that the distrust sowed by this failure has in some cases led to political extremism and even violence.

This is not the first time in American history that public health has played a major role in formulating and reinforcing political ideology. In his book *The Contagion of Liberty*, Andrew Wehrman argues that debates over smallpox inoculation represented a kind of microcosm of larger debates about liberty as the colonies attempted to gain freedom from Britain. The battle about smallpox inoculation was fought alongside the Revolution and they were intimately intertwined. In Wehrman's view, this twin battle created an early perception that disease prevention was the duty of the government. In other words, the founding of the country was marked by the notion that the government has an obligation to protect American citizens from disease.[37(p7)] Inoculation was a community-based affair, with trust at the very center—both trust of other citizens and trust of the government to ensure that inoculation campaigns were safe for everyone.[37(p319)] The following quote from the book should be read with the U.S. response to COVID-19 in mind:

> For ordinary Americans, inoculation compelled the same sacrifices and the same common commitments that winning the Revolution required. In newspaper debates, town meetings, and sometimes the deafening shouts from an incensed mob, inoculation and independence both demanded an insistence on shared burdens, an unwavering commitment to fairness, and a deep suspicion of individual ambitions and undue profit. Within those heated arguments, ordinary Americans discovered that their ideal

government was an energetic one that responded quickly to preserve the lives of all people and in the process generated both public trust and public health.[37(p319)]

If Wehrman's argument is correct, and it is quite compelling, then the United States' failure to either predict or successfully contain the COVID-19 pandemic represents a failure of the government so fundamental that it goes all the way back to expectations formed during the very founding of the country itself.

If we therefore accept the notion that public health (and trust in it) is fundamentally intertwined with trust in the government and the overall sense that the government is fulfilling its role (or not), then it would make sense that in the face of such deep distrust of the public health system, many citizens' trust in democracy itself might need to be restored. For one thing, it is very clear that vast inequities and inequalities in our society need to be remedied in order for a sense of democracy, which may never have existed for some portions of the population, to be restored. It has always been the case that extremist politics are most appealing to those who suffer while the rest of the economy grows, which defines a portion of the population that may have been abandoned by the healthcare and social safety net.[38] Plenty of research also shows that high levels of inequality lead to violence and loss of social cohesion.[38] Some have argued that our democracy has never been that secure, in part because all of the "rights" that are supposedly available to all citizens are completely circumscribed by social and political circumstances. As a result, different people experience American democracy quite differently, and some have never had faith in our country's "democratic" legacy.[39–41]

As Jonathan Manthorpe argues in *Restoring Democracy in an Age of Populists and Pestilence*, there has been an ongoing battle in America ever since the Revolutionary War about whether this country should be a true democracy or a republic governed by an economic and intellectual elite.[42(p130)] We could very clearly see this tension still at play in Trump's campaign for the presidency in 2016, in which he regularly promised to "drain the swamp," or, in other words, to rid politics of its careerist, elite figures and return power to the people. Without realizing it (most likely), Trump was pulling on the thread of a fundamental tension that has been alive and well in this country since 1776. By posing as the leader of the people, Trump fashioned himself as a defender of true democracy and a rejection of everything elitist about U.S. politics. Despite the title of his book, Manthorpe argues that Trump is not actually a populist in the truest sense of the term. Instead, in Manthrope's view, Trump's ascendancy was a product of a broken political system and a divided nation.[42(p112)] Manthorpe discusses figures such as Victor Orbán of Hungary and Andrzej Duda of Poland as true populists, whereas someone like Trump, while still espousing many populist-style views, may be more of a reflection of a political moment than someone explicitly pushing certain political ideologies. Even so, Orbán's rise to power utilizing rural Hungarians' disenchantment with urban elites certainly mirrors the circumstances around Trump's ascendancy.[42(p112)]

While it can be difficult to think of remedies to such an extreme political situation, it is worth pointing out a few possibilities. One is perhaps changing people's perceptions of what "government" is. When people think of government, their minds usually gravitate toward politics. Politics in this country right now is a bitter affair, marked by extreme partisanship and potent ingroup/outgroup sentiment. While politics may be in some ways at the center of government, it is true that government bodies do take actions that may have very little to do with politics. Social programs, especially at the state and local levels, from which many people benefit, might be one way to draw people's attention to some of the positive aspects of government even as they see a drama unfolding before them on the stage of politics.

In addition, while it may seem futile to many to do this, we do need to work harder to get behind the psychology of working-class members of American society who often say they feel like strangers in their own land, who are still recovering from the 2008 recession, in which many people in this segment of society lost their jobs or had their jobs outsourced, and now we are in another recession in part due to a failure to respond promptly and appropriately to the COVID-19 pandemic. People who never knew what a social safety net was before now find themselves in food lines. We know that people who feel more vulnerable in some way are more likely to be susceptible to the allure of extremist leaders.[43-46] We must better understand how an entire class of our society became so disillusioned that they are willing to stand up for a leader who promotes violence as a means to achieving desired political gains. I hope that I have been able to do some of this work in this book by examining how failures of the social safety net, and healthcare in particular, have turned people away from faith in the government and our democracy as they stand today. Nevertheless, I think we still have a long way to go in not only understanding this psychology, but also establishing methods to counteract associated tendencies toward extremist political ideologies.

In the immediate wake of the COVID-19 pandemic, trust in leaders and in governments was initially quite high, mostly because many leaders were following sage advice about restrictions needed to contain the spread of the disease.[42(p287)] Everything started to break down once it was time to debate lifting the restrictions. Most people saw that once states put emergency restrictions in place, they are hesitant to lift them.[42(p287)] The battle quickly became partisan and bitter, with simple behaviors such as masking becoming signals of political allegiance. This could have been a moment to come to terms with decades of social change, including high levels of migration and increasing separation between the super rich and everyone else in American society.[42(p287)] Instead, people fought, tethered themselves to conspiracy theories, and used a stressful moment to, in some cases, discover extreme political ideas that simply further divided the country.

Unfortunately, I think we might have another opportunity. COVID-19 might be receding, at least from the public policy stage, but the next pandemic is probably not that far behind. How we handle that one will once again tell us everything about how healthy or unwell our "democratic" society is. When this inevitable event occurs, perhaps a greater understanding across the population about the social forces that drive disillusionment, extreme political views, and, of course, mistrust and conspiracy theories will help bridge the bitter divide among ordinary American citizens.

Perhaps it feels like we are ending a long way off from where we started. How can a book that starts with a description of someone's distrust in doctors and medicine end on a note about the health and well-being of our democratic society? What does one have to do with the other? As I have tried to argue throughout this book, when it comes to healthcare, the economy, and the trust people have in our governmental and political institutions, everything is connected. Massive losses of trust in the healthcare system are not without consequences for the functioning of the entire government. The government is both a major provider of healthcare, even in this country, and, what's more, people actually expect the government to protect their basic well-being. When this promise is broken due to rancorous infighting, spotty access (at best) to healthcare, and soaring costs that bring people into states of true despair, it should be little surprise that the functioning of the entire democratic enterprise is in jeopardy.

This is not to say that the situation is hopeless. Small reforms and understanding by people like those reading this book can make a difference. And of course, the "small," often remarkable interventions being done at the family level make a real difference in people's lives and should be further studied and adapted on a larger scale. Our ailing nation does not have to ail. Modern medicine has met quite a challenge, but the solution lies in part in every effort that each of us takes to understand, console, and gently nudge those who feel most stuck in its crosshairs. I know I have not seen the last of email messages describing a close family member who literally died from distrust of the healthcare enterprise. But I am hoping that little by little, these stories will start to vanish. As is a common belief in the health and medical fields, there is always hope.

References

Introduction

1. Baker DW. Trust in health care in the time of COVID-19. *JAMA.* 2020;*324*(23):2373–2375. doi:10.1001/jama.2020.23343.
2. Pollard MS, Davis LM. Decline in trust in the Centers for Disease Control and Prevention during the COVID-19 pandemic. *RAND.* 2021; https://doi.org/10.7249/RRA308-12.
3. Barry C, Han H, McGinty B. *Trust in science and COVID-19.* Johns Hopkins Bloomberg School of Public Health. 2021; https://publichealth.jhu.edu/2020/trust-in-science-and-covid-19
4. ABIM Foundation, NORC. *Surveys of trust in the U.S. healthcare system.* 2021. https://www.norc.org/content/dam/norc-org/pdfs/20210514_NORC_ABIM_Foundation_Trust%20in%20Healthcare_FINAL.pdf
5. Bogart LM, Ojikutu BO, Tyagi K, et al. COVID-19 related medical mistrust, health impacts, and potential vaccine hesitancy among Black Americans living with HIV. *J Acquir Immune Defic Syndr.* 2021;*86*(2):200–207.
6. Choi Y, Fox AM. Mistrust in public health institutions is a stronger predictor of vaccine hesitancy and uptake than trust in Trump. *Soc Sci Med.* 2022;*314*:115440. doi:https://doi.org/10.1016/j.socscimed.2022.115440.
7. Baumgaertner B, Carlisle JE, Justwan F. The influence of political ideology and trust on willingness to vaccinate. *PLoS ONE.* 2018;*13*:e0191728.
8. Callaghan T, Moghtaderi A, Lueck JA, et al. Correlates and disparities of intention to vaccinate against COVID-19. *Soc Sci Med.* 2021;*272*:113638.
9. Jamison AM, Quinna SC, Freimuth VS. "You don't trust a government vaccine": narratives of institutional trust and influenza vaccination among African American and White adults. *Soc Sci Med.* 2019;*221*:87–94.
10. Merkley E, Loewen PJ. Anti-intellectualism and the mass public's response to the COVID-19 pandemic. *Nat Hum Behav.* 2021;*5*:706–715.
11. Taylor S, Asmundson GJG. Negative attitudes about facemasks during the COVID-19 pandemic: the dual importance of perceived ineffectiveness and psychological reactance. *PLoS ONE.* 2021;*16*(2):e0246317. https://doi.org/10.1371/journal.pone.0246317.
12. Commonwealth Fund. *Mirror, Mirror 2021: Reflecting Poorly,* 2021. New York: Commonwealth Fund. https://www.commonwealthfund.org/publications/fund-reports/2021/aug/mirror-mirror-2021-reflecting-poorly.
13. National Center for Health Statistics. *Health Insurance Coverage: Early Release of Estimates from the National Health Interview Survey, 2021.* Washington, DC: U.S. Department of Health & Human Services & CDC; 2022. https://www.cdc.gov/nchs/data/nhis/earlyrelease/insur202205.pd.f
14. Conger K. How misinformation, medical mistrust fuel vaccine hesitancy. *Stanford Med.* 2021. https://med.stanford.edu/news/all-news/2021/09/infodemic-covid-19.html.
15. Khullar D, Darien G, Ness DL. Patient consumerism, healing relationships, and rebuilding trust in health care. *JAMA.* 2020;*324*(23):2359–2360.
16. Brown KV. Why one woman's family began drinking bleach. *Bloomberg.* 2023. https://www.bloomberg.com/news/newsletters/2023-03-15/why-one-woman-s-family-began-drinking-bleach.

17. Hyacinthe M, Whittaker S. Vaccine hesitancy and medical mistrust: what did we learn? *Interdisciplinary Association of Population Health Sciences.* https://iaphs.org/vaccine-hesitancy-and-medical-mistrust-what-did-we-learn/.

18. Ray R, Rojas F. COVID-19 and the future of society. *Contexts.* 2020. https://contexts.org/blog/covid-19-and-the-future-of-society/#hyde.

19. Leonard MB, Pursley DM, Robinson LA, et al. The importance of trustworthiness: lessons from the COVID-19 pandemic. *Pediatr Res.* 2022;*91*:482–485; https://doi.org/10.1038/s41390-021-01866-z.

20. Romer D, Jamieson KH. Patterns of media use, strength of belief in COVID-19 conspiracy theories, and the prevention of COVID-19 from March to July 2020 in the United States: survey study. *J Med Internet Res.* 2021;*23*(4):e25215. doi:10.2196/25215.

21. Quinn EK, Fazel SS, Peters CE. The Instagram infodemic: cobranding of conspiracy theories, coronavirus disease 2019 and authority-questioning beliefs. *Cyberpsychology Behav Soc Netw.* 2021;*24*(8):573–577. http://doi.org/10.1089/cyber.2020.0663.

22. Pavela BI, Banai B, Mikloušić I. Beliefs in covid-19 conspiracy theories, compliance with the preventive measures, and trust in government medical officials. *Curr Psychol.* 2021;*41*(10):7448–7458. https://doi.org/10.1007/s12144-021-01898-y.

23. Uscinski JE, Enders AM. The coronavirus conspiracy boom. *The Atlantic.* 2020; https://www.theatlantic.com/health/archive/2020/04/what-can-coronavirus-tell-us-about-conspiracy-theories/610894/.

24. Romer D, Jamieson KH. Conspiracy theories as barriers to controlling the spread of COVID-19 in the U.S. *Soc Sci Med.* 2020;*263*:113356. http://dx.doi.org/10.1016/j.socscimed.2020.113356.

25. Earnshaw VA, Eaton LA, Kalichman SC, et al. COVID-19 conspiracy beliefs, health behaviors, and policy support. *TBM.* 2020;*10*:850–856. doi:10.1093/tbm/ibaa090.

26. Brown K, Mondon A, Winter A. The far right, the mainstream and mainstreaming: towards a heuristic framework. *J Polit Ideol.* 2023;*28*(2):162–179.

27. Schain MA. Shifting tides: radical right populism and immigration policy in Europe and the United States. *Migration Policy Institute.* 2018; https://www.migrationpolicy.org/sites/default/files/publications/Schain-PopulismUSandEurope-Final-Web.pdf.

28. Jones SG. The rise of far-right extremism in the United States. *Center for Strategic & International Studies.* 2018; https://csis-website-prod.s3.amazonaws.com/s3fs-public/publication/181119_RightWingTerrorism_layout_FINAL.pdf?MyC9DjLLRftoeUKvq6qxFPsCPFoTkBpH.

29. Assessing threats of political violence and rising extremism on the far-right. *PBS Newshour.* 2022; https://www.pbs.org/newshour/show/assessing-rising-extremism-on-the-right.

30. Kleinfeld R. The rise of political violence in the United States. *J Democr.* 2021;*32*(4):160–176.

31. Miller-Idriss, C. How extremism went mainstream. *Foreign Aff.* January 3, 2022; https://www.foreignaffairs.com/articles/united-states/2022-01-03/how-extremism-went-mainstream.

32. Greven T. *The Rise of Right-Wing Populism in Europe and the United States.* New York: Friedrich Ebert Stiftung; 2016.

Chapter 1

1. Blendon RJ, Benson JM, Hero JA. Public trust in physicians: U.S. medicine in international perspective. *N Engl J Med.* 2014;*371*:1570–1572.

2. Norman J. Americans' confidence in institutions stays low. *Gallup.* 2016; https://news.gallup.com/poll/192581/americans-confidence-institutions-stays-low.aspx.

3. Doherty C, Kiley J, Asheer N, Jordan C. Americans' views of government: low trust, but some positive performance ratings. *Pew Research Center.* 2020; https://www.pewresearch.

org/politics/2020/09/14/americans-views-of-government-low-trust-but-some-positive-performance-ratings/.

4. Simione L, Vagni M, Gnagnarella C, Bersani G, Pajardi D. Mistrust and beliefs in conspiracy theories differently mediate the effects of psychological factors on propensity for COVID-19 Vaccine. *Front Psychol.* 2021;*12*:683–684.

5. Jennings W, Stoker G, Bunting H, et al. Lack of trust, conspiracy beliefs, and social media use predict COVID-19 vaccine hesitancy. *Vaccines.* 2021;*9*(6):593.

6. Roozenbeek J, Schneider CR, Dryhurst S, et al. Susceptibility to misinformation about COVID-19 around the world. *R Soc Open Sci.* 2020;*7*:201199.

7. Gorman JM, Gorman SE, Sandy W, et al. Implications of COVID-19 vaccine hesitancy: results of online bulletin board interviews. *Front Public Health.* 2022;*9*:757283. https://doi.org/10.3389/fpubh.2021.757283.

8. James C. Mistrust is the biggest health crisis facing the United States today. *Grantmakers in Health.* 2021; https://www.gih.org/from-the-president/mistrust-is-the-biggest-health-crisis-facing-the-united-states-today/.

9. Khullar D. Do you trust the medical profession? *New York Times. January 23,* 2018; https://www.nytimes.com/2018/01/23/upshot/do-you-trust-the-medical-profession.html.

10. Corbin I, Waters J. U.S. health care faces a crisis of trust. *Newsweek.* 2021; https://www.newsweek.com/us-health-care-faces-crisis-trust-opinion-1635658.

11. Schaeffer K. A look at the Americans who believe there is some truth to the conspiracy theory that COVID-19 was planned. *Pew Research Center.* 2020; https://www.pewresearch.org/short-reads/2020/07/24/a-look-at-the-americans-who-believe-there-is-some-truth-to-the-conspiracy-theory-that-covid-19-was-planned/.

12. Merlan A. *Republic of Lies: American Conspiracy Theorists and Their Surprising Rise to Power.* New York: Metropolitan Books; 2019.

13. Cassam Q. *Conspiracy Theories.* Cambridge, UK: Polity; 2019.

14. Baron R. The dangers of mistrust in healthcare. *Aspen Institute.* 2019; https://www.aspeninstitute.org/blog-posts/the-danger-of-mistrust-in-health-care/.

15. Americans distrust government, but want it to do more. *Kaiser Family Foundation.* 2019; https://www.kff.org/wp-content/uploads/2013/01/americans-trust-government-but-want-it-to-do-more.pdf.

16. Funk C, Gramlich J. Amid coronavirus threat, Americans generally have a high level of trust in medical doctors. *Pew Research Center.* 2020; https://www.pewresearch.org/fact-tank/2020/03/13/amid-coronavirus-threat-americans-generally-have-a-high-level-of-trust-in-medical-doctors/.

17. Funk C, Hefferon M, Kennedy B, Johnson C. Trust and mistrust in Americans' views of scientific experts. *Pew Research Center.* 2019; https://www.pewresearch.org/science/2019/08/02/trust-and-mistrust-in-americans-views-of-scientific-experts/.

18. Haefner M. COVID-19 shifts Americans' view of physicians: 5 things to know. *Becker's Hospital Review.* 2020; https://www.beckershospitalreview.com/strategy/covid-19-shifts-americans-view-of-physicians-5-things-to-know.html.

19. 75% of U.S. consumers wish their healthcare experiences were more personalized. *Business Wire.* 2020; https://www.businesswire.com/news/home/20200218005006/en/75-of-U.S.-Consumers-Wish-Their-Healthcare-Experiences-Were-More-Personalized-Redpoint-Global-Survey-Reveals.

20. Surveys of trust in the U.S. health care system. ABIM Foundation, NORC at the University of Chicago. 2021; https://www.norc.org/PDFs/ABIM%20Foundation/20210520_NORC_ABIM_Foundation_Trust%20in%20Healthcare_Part%201.pdf.

21. Bach RL, Wenz A. Studying health-related internet and mobile device use using weblogs and smartphone records. *PLoS ONE.* 2021;*15*(6):e0234663.

22. Bekker HL, Winterbottom AE, Butow P, et al. Do personal stories make patient decision aids more effective? A critical review of theory and evidence. *BMC Med Inform Decis Mak.* 2013;*13*(2):S9.

23. Dohan D, Garrett SB, Rendle KA. The importance of integrating narrative into health care decision making. *Health Aff.* 2016;*35*(4):720–725.

24. Newport F. Most Americans take doctor's advice without second opinion. *Gallup News.* 2010; https://news.gallup.com/poll/145025/americans-doctor-advice-without-second-opinion.aspx.

25. Fox S. What ails America? Dr. Google can tell you. *Pew Research Center.* 2013; https://www.pewresearch.org/fact-tank/2013/12/17/what-ails-america-dr-google-can-tell-you/.

26. Huang EC, Pu C, Chou Y, Huang N. Public trust in physicians–health care commodification as a possible deteriorating factor: cross-sectional analysis of 23 countries. *Inquiry.* 2018;*55*:46958018759174.

27. Halpern SD, Loewenstein G, Volpp KG. Default options in advance directives influence how patients set goals for end-of-life care. *Health Aff.* 2013;*32*(2):408–417.

28. Johnson EJ. We only think we're making our own choices. It matters how options are framed. *TIME.* 2021; https://time.com/6114884/how-we-make-decisions-with-choice-architecture/.

29. Chubak B. Clinical responsibility in the age of patient autonomy. *Virtual Mentor.* 2009;*11*(8):567–570.

30. Kilbride MK, Joffe S. The new age of patient autonomy: implications for the patient-physician relationship. *JAMA.* 2018;*320*(19):1973–1974.

31. Bardon A. *The Truth About Denial: Bias and Self-Deception in Science, Politics, and Religion.* Oxford: Oxford University Press; 2019.

32. Kunda Z. The case for motivated reasoning. *Psychol Bull.* 1990;*108*(3):480–498.

33. Kahan D. Ideology, motivated reasoning, and cognitive reflection. *Judgm Decis Mak.* 2013;*8*(4):407–424.

34. Epley N, Gilovich T. The mechanics of motivated reasoning. *J Econ Perspect.* 2016;*30*(3):133–140.

35. Shapiro JP. The thinking error at the root of science denial. *The Conversation.* 2018; https://theconversation.com/the-thinking-error-at-the-root-of-science-denial-96099.

36. Sturgis P, Brunton-Smith I, Jackson J. Trust in science, social consensus, and vaccine confidence. *Nat Hum Behav.* 2021;*5*:1528–1534.

37. Brzezinski A, Kecht V, Van Dijcke D, Wright AL. Science skepticism reduced compliance with COVID-19 shelter-in-place policies in the United States. *Nat Hum Behav.* 2021;*5*:1519–1527.

38. Merkley E, Loewen PJ. Anti-intellectualism and the mass public's response to the COVID-19 pandemic. *Nat Hum Behav.* 2021;*5*:706–715.

39. Henderson J, Ward PR, Tonkin E, et al. Developing and maintaining public trust during and post-COVID-19: can we apply a model developed for responding to food scares? *Front Public Health.* 2020;*8*:369.

40. Clinical practice guidelines we can trust. *Institute of Medicine.* 2011; https://www.nap.edu/catalog/13058/clinical-practice-guidelines-we-can-trust.

41. Rainie L, Keeter S, Perrin A. Trust and distrust in America. *Pew Research Center.* 2019; https://www.pewresearch.org/politics/2019/07/22/how-americans-see-problems-of-trust/.

42. Borsari B, Carey KB. Descriptive and injunctive norms in college drinking: a meta-analytic integration. *J Stud Alcohol.* 2003;*64*(3):331–341.

43. Pennycook G, Epstein Z, Mosleh M, Arechar AA, Eckles D, Rand DG. Shifting attention to accuracy can reduce misinformation online. *Nature.* 2021;*592*:590–595.

44. van der Linden S, Leiserowitz A, Rosenthal S, Maibach E. Inoculating the public against misinformation about climate change. *Global Chall.* 2017;*1*(2):1600008.

45. Banas JA, Rains SA. A meta-analysis of research on inoculation theory. *Commun Monog.* 2010;*77*(3):281–311.

46. Tanaka Y, Hirayama R. Exposure to countering messages online: alleviating or strengthening false belief? *Cyberpsychol Behav Soc Netw.* 2019;*22*(11):742–746.

47. Pennycook G, Bear A, Collins ET, Rand DG. The implied truth effect: attaching warnings to a subset of fake news stories increases perceived accuracy of stories without warnings. *Researchgate.net.* 2017; https://www.researchgate.net/profile/Gordon_Pennycook/publ ication/321887941_The_Implied_Truth_Effect_Attaching_warnings_to_a_subset_of_ fake_news_stories_increases_perceived_accuracy_of _stories_without_warnings/links/ 5caacda34585157bd32a69b3/The-Implied-Truth-Effect-Attachingwarnings-to-a-subset- of-fake-news-stories-increases-perceived-accuracy-of-stories-withoutwarnings.pdf.

48. Clayton K, Blair S, Busam JA, et al. Real solutions for fake news? Measuring the effective- ness of general warnings and fact-check tags in reducing belief in false stories on social media. *Polit Behav.* 2020;*42*:1073–1095.

49. Ecker UKH, Lewandowsky S, Tang DTW. Explicit warnings reduce but do not eliminate the continued influence of misinformation. *Mem Cogn.* 2010;*38*(8):1087–1100.

50. Bronstein MV, Pennycook G, Bear A, Rand DG. Belief in fake news is associated with delusionality, dogmatism, religious fundamentalism, and reduced analytic thinking. *J Appl Res Mem Cogn.* 2019;*8*(1):108–117.

51. Martel C, Pennycook G, Rand D. Reliance on emotion promotes belief in fake news. *Psyarxiv.com.* 2019. https://psyarxiv.com/a2ydw/.

52. Pennycook G, Cheyne JA, Koehler D, Fugelsang JA. On the belief that beliefs should change according to evidence: implications for conspiratorial, moral, paranormal, polit- ical, religious, and science beliefs. Psyarxiv.com. https://psyarxiv.com/a7k96/download/ ?format=pdf.

53. Pennycook G, Rand DG. Lazy, not biased: susceptibility to partisan fake news is better explained by lack of reasoning than by motivated reasoning. *Cognition.* 2019;*188*: 39–50.

54. Miller WR. Motivational interviewing with problem drinkers. *Behav Psychother.* 1983;*11*:147–172.

55. Reims KG, Ernst D. Using motivational interviewing to promote healthy weight. *FPM.* 2016;*23*(5):32–38.

56. Lindson N, Thompson TP, Ferrey A, Lambert JD, Aveyard P. Motivational interviewing for smoking cessation. *Cochrane Database Syst Rev.* 2019;*7*(7):CD006936.

57. Bandura A. Self-efficacy: toward a unifying theory of behavioral change. *Psychol Rev.* 1977;*84*:191–215.

58. Rabin RC. Overdose deaths reached record high as the pandemic spread. *New York Times. November 17,* 2021; https://www.nytimes.com/2021/11/17/health/drug-overdoses-fenta nyl-deaths.html.

59. Kahan DM, Landrum A, Carpenter K, Helft L, Jamieson KH. Science curiosity and polit- ical information processing. *Polit Psychol.* 2017;*38*(1).

60. Jirout JJ. Supporting early scientific thinking through curiosity. *Front Psychol.* 2020;*11*:1717.

61. Eichmeier LA, Stenhouse N. Reducing motivated reasoning on controversial sci- ence: testing which factors best promote open-minded processing of information. PCST Network. 2018. https://pcst.co/archive/conference/paper/351.

62. Gaither SE, Fan SP, Kinzler KD. Thinking about multiple identities boosts children's flex- ible thinking. *Dev Sci.* 2019;*23*(1):e0012871.

Chapter 2

1. Miller F, Miller P. Transgenerational trauma and trust restoration. *AMA J Ethics.* 2021;*23*(6):E480–E486.

2. Williams JC. Black Americans don't trust our healthcare system—here's why. *The Hill.* 2017; https://thehill.com/blogs/pundits-blog/healthcare/347780-black-americans-dont- have-trust-in-our-healthcare-system/.

3. Royles D. Years of medical abuse make Black Americans less likely to trust the Coronavirus vaccine. *Washington Post*. December 15, 2020; https://www.washingtonpost.com/outl ook/2020/12/15/years-medical-abuse-make-black-americans-less-likely-trust-covid-vaccine/.

4. Roberts J. African American belief narratives and the African cultural tradition. *Res African Lit*. 2009;*40*(1):112–126.

5. Alsan M, Wanamaker M. Tuskegee and the health of Black Men. *Q J Economics*. 2018;*133*(1):407–455.

6. Hall OT, Bhadra-Heintz NM, Teater J, et al. Group-based medical mistrust and care expectations among Black patients seeking addiction treatment. *Drug Alcohol Depend*. 2021;*2*:100026.

7. Balasuriya L, Santilli A, Morone J, et al. COVID-19 vaccine acceptance and access among Black and Latinx communities. *JAMA Network Open*. 2021;*4*(10):e2128575.

8. Washington HA. *Medical Apartheid: The Dark History of Medical Experimentation on Black Americans from Colonial Times to the Present*. New York: Doubleday; 2006.

9. Associated Press. Amid Coronavirus pandemic, Black mistrust of medicine looms. *Mod Healthc*. 2020; https://www.modernhealthcare.com/patient-care/amid-coronavirus-pande mic-black-mistrust-medicine-looms.

10. Gamble VN. Under the shadow of Tuskegee: African Americans and health care. *Am J Public Health*. 1997;*87*(11):1773–1778.

11. Hahmed S, Bradby H, Ahlberg BM. Racism in healthcare: a scoping review. *BMC Public Health*. 2022;*22*(988).

12. Feagin J, Bennefield Z. Systemic racism and U.S. health care. *Soc Sci Med*. 2014;*103*:7–14.

13. Byrd WM, Clayton LA. Race, medicine, and health care in the United States: a historical survey. *J Natl Med Assoc*. 2001;*93*(3):11S–34S.

14. Williams DR, Lawrence J, Davis B. Racism and health: evidence and needed research. *Ann Rev Public Health*. 2019;*40*:105–125.

15. Alcindor Y, Wellford R, Lloyd B, Bolaji L. With a history of abuse in American medicine, Black patients struggle for equal access. *PBS Newshour*. 2021; https://www.pbs.org/newsh our/show/with-a-history-of-abuse-in-american-medicine-black-patients-struggle-for-equal-access.

16. Dembosky A. It's not Tuskegee: current medical racism fuels Black Americans' vaccine hesitancy. *LA Times*. March 25, 2021; https://www.latimes.com/science/story/2021-03-25/ current-medical-racism-not-tuskegee-expls-vaccine-hesitancy-among-black-americans.

17. Barzagan M, Cobb S, Assari S. Discrimination and medical mistrust in a racially and ethnically diverse sample of California adults. *Ann Fam Med*. 2021;*19*(1):4–15.

18. Benkert R, Peters RM, Templin TN. Sociodemographics and medical mistrust in a population based sample of Michigan residents. *Int J Nurs Health Care Res*. 2019;*6*:092.

19. Do YK, Carpenter WR, Spain P, et al. Race, healthcare access and physician trust among prostate cancer patients. *Cancer Causes Control*. 2010;*21*(1):31–40.

20. Weech-Maldonado R, Hall A, Bryant T, Jenkins KA, Elliott MN. The relationship between perceived discrimination and patient experiences with health care. *Med Care*. 2012;*50*(9 Suppl 2):S62–S68.

21. Duke CC, Stanik C. Overcoming lower income patients' concerns about trust and respect from providers. *Health Aff Forefront*. 2016; https://www.healthaffairs.org/do/10.1377/ forefront.20160811.056138/full/.

22. Becker, G., Newsom, E. Socioeconomic status and dissatisfaction with health care among chronically ill African Americans. *Am J Public Health*. 2003;*93*(5):742–748.

23. Himmelstein G, Bates D, Zhou L. Examination of stigmatizing language in the electronic health record. *JAMA Open Network*. 2022;*5*(1):e2144967.

24. Sun M, Oliwa T, Peek ME, et al. Negative patient descriptors: documenting racial bias in the electronic health record. *Health Aff*. 2022;*41*(2):203–211.

25. Myers JR, Ball K, Jeffers SL. Medical Mmistrust, HIV-related conspiracy beliefs, and the need for cognitive closure among urban-residing African American women: an exploratory study. *J Health Disparities Res Pract.* 2018;*11*(4):138–148.

26. Powell W, Richmond J, Mohottige D, et al. Medical mistrust, racism, and delays in preventive health screening among African-American men. *Behav Med.* 2019;*45*(2):102–117.

27. Smith AC, Woerner J, Perera R, et al. An investigation of associations between race, ethnicity, and past experiences of discrimination with medical mistrust and COVID-19 protective strategies. *J Racial Ethn Health Disparities.* 2021;*9*:1430–1442.

28. Hamel L, Lopes L, Munana C, et al. *Race, Health, and COVID-19: The Views and Experiences of Black Americans.* San Francisco: Kaiser Family Foundation; 2020.

29. Funk C, Kennedy B, Johnson C. *Trust in medical scientists has grown in U.S., but mainly among democrats.* Pew Research Center; 2020. https://www.pewresearch.org/science/2020/05/21/trust-in-medical-scientists-has-grown-in-u-s-but-mainly-among-democrats/

30. Byrd WM, Clayton LA. *An American Health Dilemma: A Medical History of African Americans and the Problem of Race.* New York: Routledge; 2000.

31. Benisek A. COVID-19 vaccines. *WebMD.* 2022; https://www.webmd.com/vaccines/covid-19-vaccine/news/20210202/black-vaccine-hesitancy-rooted-in-mistrust-doubts.

32. Yuko E. Why are Black communities being singled out as vaccine hesitant? *Rolling Stone.* 2021; https://www.rollingstone.com/culture/culture-features/covid-19-vaccine-hesitant-black-communities-singled-out-1137750/.

34. Khubchandani J, Macias Y. COVID-19 vaccination hesitancy in Hispanics and African-Americans: a review and recommendations for practice. *Brain Behav Immun Health.* 2021;*15*:100277.

35. Hamel L, Kirzinger A, Lopes L, et al. KFF COVID-19 Vaccine monitor: January 2021. *Kaiser Family Foundation.* 2021; https://www.kff.org/coronavirus-covid-19/report/kff-covid-19-vaccine-monitor-january-2021/.

36. Mochkofsky G. The Latinx community and COVID-disinformation campaigns. *The New Yorker.* 2022; https://www.newyorker.com/news/daily-comment/the-latinx-community-and-covid-disinformation-campaigns.

37. Garcia J, Vargas N, de la Torre C, et al. Engaging Latino families about COVID-19 vaccines: a qualitative study conducted in Oregon, USA. *Health Educ Behav.* 2021;*48*(6):747–757.

38. Jaiswal J, Halkitis PN. Towards a more inclusive and dynamic understanding of medical mistrust informed by science. *Behav Med.* 2019;*45*(2):79–85.

39. Leon B. Many Latinos are hesitant to get a COVID-19 vaccine. *NPR.* 2021; https://www.npr.org/2021/02/01/962905232/many-latinos-are-hesitant-to-get-a-covid-19-vaccine.

40. Rodriguez MA, Garcia R. First, do no harm: the US sexually transmitted disease experiments in Guatemala. *Am J Public Health.* 2013;*103*(12):2122–2126.

41. Kricorian K, Turner K. COVID-19 vaccine acceptance and beliefs among Black and Hispanic Americans. *PLoS ONE.* 2021;*16*(8):e0256122.

42. Sakran JV, Hilton EJ, Sathya C. Racism in health care isn't always obvious. *Sci Am.* 2020; https://www.scientificamerican.com/article/racism-in-health-care-isnt-always-obvious/.

43. Ollove M. With implicit bias hurting patients, some states train doctors. *Pew.* 2022; https://www.pewtrusts.org/en/research-and-analysis/blogs/stateline/2022/04/21/with-implicit-bias-hurting-patients-some-states-train-doctors.

44. Alsan M, Garrick O, Graziani GC. *Does Diversity Matter for Health? Experimental Evidence from Oakland. National Bureau of Economic Research;* 2018.

45. Horne C, Kennedy EH. The power of social norms for reducing and shifting electricity use. *Energy Policy.* 2017;*107*:43–52.

46. Bonan J, Cattaneo C, d'Adda G, Tavoni M. The interaction of descriptive and injunctive social norms in promoting energy conservation. *Nature Energy.* 2020;*5*:900–909.

47. Schultz PW, Nolan JM, Cialdini RB, et al. The constructive, destructive, and reconstructive power of social norms. *Psychol Sci.* 2007;*18*(5):429–434.

48. Stonko DP, Dun C, Walsh CW, et al. Evaluation of a physician peer-benchmarking intervention for practice variability and costs for endovenous thermal ablation. *JAMA Network Open.* 2021;4(12):e2137515.

49. Meeker D, Friedberg MW, Knight TK, et al. Effect of peer benchmarking on specialist electronic consult performance in a Los Angeles safety net: a cluster randomized trial. *J Gen Intern Med.* 2021;37:1400–1407.

50. Albertini JG, Wang P, Fahim C, et al. Evaluation of a peer-to-peer data transparency intervention for Mohs micrographic surgery overuse. *JAMA Dermatol.* 2019;155(8):906–913.

51. Meeker D, Linder JA, Fox CR. Effect of behavioral interventions on inappropriate antibiotic prescribing among primary care practices: a randomized clinical trial. *JAMA.* 2016;315(6):562–570.

52. Francois A, Johnson SL, Waasdorp TE, et al. Association between adolescents' perceptions of alcohol norms and alcohol behaviors: incorporating within-school variability. *Am J Health Educ.* 2017;48(2):80–89.

53. Pederson ER, Osilla KC, Miles JNV, et al. The role of perceived injunctive alcohol norms in adolescent drinking behavior. *Addict Behav.* 2017;67:1–7.

54. Bogart LM, Dong L, Gandhi P, et al. *What Contributes to COVID-19 Vaccine Hesitancy in Black Communities, and How Can it Be Addressed? RAND;* 2022.

Chapter 3

1. Ferguson Z, Kelsey-Sugg A. COVID conspiracies are just the latest theories in a history stretching back centuries. *Australian Broadcasting Corporation.* 2022; https://www.abc.net.au/news/2022-01-11/medical-conspiracies-a-history-from-covid-back-to-ancient-rome/100672978.

2. Rothschild M. *The Storm Is Upon Us: How QAnon Became a Movement, Cult, and Conspiracy Theory of Everything.* New York: Melville House; 2021.

3. Pertwee E, Simas C, Larson HJ. An epidemic of uncertainty: rumors, conspiracy theories and vaccine hesitancy. *Nat Med.* 2022;28:456–459.

4. Fassin D. Conspiracy theories as crisis and critique. *Moose Lecture.* June 10, 2021; https://www.youtube.com/watch?v=HCfKys4uUQE.

5. Carey B. A theory about conspiracy theories. *New York Times. September 28,* 2020; https://www.nytimes.com/2020/09/28/health/psychology-conspiracy-theories.html.

6. Shute N. Half of Americans believe in medical conspiracy theories. *NPR.* 2014; https://www.npr.org/sections/health-shots/2014/03/19/291405689/half-of-americans-believe-in-medical-conspiracy-theories.

7. Oliver JE, Wood T. Medical conspiracy theories and health behaviors in the United States. *JAMA Intern Med.* 2014;174(5):817–818.

8. Van der Linden S, Panagopoulos C, Azevedo F. The paranoid style in American politics revisited: an ideological asymmetry in conspiratorial thinking. *Polit Psychol.* 2020;42(1):23–51.

9. Pierre JM. Mistrust and misinformation: a two-component, socio-epistemic model of belief in conspiracy theories. *J Soc Polit Psychol.* 2020;8(2):617–641.

10. Johns Hopkins Medicine. Mental health disorder statistics; https://www.hopkinsmedicine.org/health/wellness-and-prevention/mental-health-disorder-statistics.

11. Oliver JE, Wood TJ. Conspiracy theories and the paranoid style(s) of mass opinion. *Am J Polit Sci.* 2014;58(4):952–966.

12. Pies RW, Pierre JM. Believing in conspiracy theories is not delusional. *Medscape.* 2021; https://www.medscape.com/viewarticle/945290.

13. van Prooijen J. *The Psychology of Conspiracy Theories (The Psychology of Everything).* New York: Routledge; 2018.

14. Cohn M. Conspiracy theories muddy Zika public health message. *Baltimore Sun. May 30,* 2016; https://www.baltimoresun.com/health/bs-hs-zika-conspiracies-20160530-story. html.

15. Shaeffer K. A look at the Americans who believe there is some truth to the conspiracy theory that COVID-19 was planned. *Pew Research Center.* 2020; https://www.pewresea rch.org/fact-tank/2020/07/24/a-look-at-the-americans-who-believe-there-is-some-truth-to-the-conspiracy-theory-that-covid-19-was-planned/.

16. Orth, T. Which groups of Americans are most likely to believe conspiracy theories. *YouGov America.* 2022; https://today.yougov.com/topics/politics/articles-reports/2022/03/30/ which-groups-americans-believe-conspiracies.

17. Newby K. *Bitten: The Secret History of Lyme Disease and Biological Weapons.* New York: Harper Wave; 2019.

18. Blaylock RL. COVID update: what is the truth? *Surg Neurol Int.* 2022;*13*:167.

19. Bodner J, Welch W, Brodie I. *COVID-19 Conspiracy Theories: QAnon, 5G, the New World Order and Other Viral Ideas.* Jefferson, NC: McFarland; 2020.

20. Greene R, Robison-Greene R. *Conspiracy Theories: Philosophers Connect the Dots.* Chicago: Open Court; 2020.

21. Uscinski JE, Enders AM, Klofstad C. Why do people believe COVID-19 conspiracy theories? *HKS Misinformation Rev.* 2020;*1*. https://doi.org/10.37016/mr-2020-015.

22. Simione L, Vagni M, Gnagnarella C, et al. Mistrust and beliefs in conspiracy theories differently mediate the effects of psychological factors on propensity for COVID-19 vaccine. *Front. Psychol.* 2021;*12*:683–684.

23. Douglas K. Why people believe in conspiracy theories. *APA Speaking of Psychology.* 2021; https://www.apa.org/news/podcasts/speaking-of-psychology/conspiracy-theories.

24. Badham V. *QAnon and On: A Short and Shocking History of the Internet Conspiracy Cults.* Melbourne: Hardie Grant Books; 2022.

25. Jamison AM, Broniatowski DA, Dredze M. not just conspiracy theories: vaccine opponents and proponents add to the COVID-19 "infodemic" on Twitter. *HKS Misinformation Rev.* 2020;*1*:1–22. https://doi.org/10.37016/mr-2020-38.

26. Drażkiewicz, E. Study conspiracy theories with compassion. *Nature.* 2022:765. https:// www.nature.com/articles/d41586-022-00879-w

27. Cirignano D. *American Conspiracies and Cover-Ups: JFK, 9/11, the Fed, Rigged Elections, Suppressed Cancer Cures, and the Greatest Conspiracies of Our Time.* New York: Skyhorse; 2019.

28. Brumfiel G. Their mom died of COVID. They say conspiracy theories are what really killed her. *NPR Shots.* 2022; https://www.npr.org/sections/health-shots/2022/04/24/108 9786147/covid-conspiracy-theories.

29. Yousef O. The "great replacement" conspiracy theory isn't fringe anymore, it's mainstream. *NPR.* 2022; https://www.nprillinois.org/2022-05-17/the-great-replacement-conspiracy-theory-isnt-fringe-anymore-its-mainstream.

30. *Fox News.* Ingraham: Coronavirus crisis is teaching us a lot about so-called experts. April 13, 2020; https://www.youtube.com/watch?v=222kvZPu7_U.

31. *Fox News.* Ingraham: Fauci "routinely" acted against science. June 10, 2021; https://www. youtube.com/watch?v=O1TA6ISXBjI.

32. *Fox News.* Ingraham: The truth behind hydroxychloroquine. April 22, 2020; https://www. youtube.com/watch?v=RexUJeWmzSE.

33. *The View.* Ted Cruz: New York, New Jersey's COVID-19 response. September 28, 2020; https://www.youtube.com/watch?v=mLvH3F17BhU.

34. *ABC News.* Sen. Ted Cruz reacts to coronavirus response, quarantine experience. March 13, 2020; https://www.youtube.com/watch?v=YtDqNNR5nxQ.

35. *Fox News.* Ted Cruz blasts Democrats' "rank hypocrisy" surrounding COVID positive migrants. July 28, 2021; https://www.youtube.com/watch?v=4JFABUkRaO0.

36. Sen. Ted Cruz on COVID vaccine mandates. *Senate Floor,* February 17, 2022; https://www.youtube.com/watch?v=dYbwXhE2Ryo.

37. Episode 61: Will we ever return to normal? Verdict with Ted Cruz, December 8, 2020; https://www.youtube.com/watch?v=2WS3tcXtdYc.

38. Nancy Pelosi, chief mask officer. *Verdict with Ted Cruz,* August 6, 2021; https://www.youtube.com/watch?v=e3yYaUcI96k.

39. *CNN.* Marjorie Taylor Greene dodges Acosta's questions in street interview. April 30, 2022; https://www.youtube.com/watch?v=q4WLiF2imfM.

40. Van Prooijen J, Etienne TW, Kutiyski Y, et al. Conspiracy beliefs prospectively predict health behavior and well-being during a pandemic. *Psychol Med.* 2021;53(6):2514–2521. https://doi.org/ 10.1017/S0033291721004438.

41. Friedman RA. Why humans are vulnerable to conspiracy theories. *Psychiatr Serv.* 2021;72(1):3–4.

Chapter 4

1. Allen D. *Democracy in the Time of Coronavirus.* Chicago: University of Chicago Press; 2022.

2. Zamarripa R. 5 ways the Trump administration's policy failures compounded the coronavirus-induced economic crisis. *Center for American Progress.* 2020; https://www.americanprogress.org/article/5-ways-trump-administrations-policy-failures-compounded-coronavirus-induced-economic-crisis/.

3. Robbins R, Garde D, Feuerstein A. An expert's take on what the U.S., U.K. did wrong in COVID-19 communications—and what others did right. *STAT.* 2020; https://www.statnews.com/2020/09/18/an-experts-take-on-what-the-u-s-u-k-did-wrong-in-covid-19-communications-and-what-others-did-right/.

4. Dickinson T. The four men responsible for America's COVID-19 test disaster. *Rolling Stone.* 2020; https://www.rollingstone.com/politics/politics-features/covid-19-test-trump-admin-failed-disaster-995930/.

5. Schneider RO. *An Unmitigated Disaster: America's Response to COVID-19.* Westport, CT: Praeger; 2022.

6. Lewis T. How the U.S. pandemic response went wrong—and what went right—during a year of COVID. *Sci Am.* 2021.

7. Feachem NS, Sander K, Barker F. The United States' response to COVID-19: a case study of the first year. *UCSF Institute for Global Health Sciences.* 2021.

8. Yong, E. How the pandemic defeated America. *The Atlantic.* September 2020.

9. Simmons-Duffin S, Huang P. A year in, experts assess Biden's hits and misses on handling the pandemic. *NPR Shots.* 2022.

10. Vinjamuri L. America's coronavirus response is shaped by its federal structure. *Chatham House.* March 2020; https://www.chathamhouse.org/2020/03/americas-coronavirus-response-shaped-its-federal-structure.

11. *NBC News.* Trump, White House Task Force hold briefing. April 13, 2020; https://www.youtube.com/watch?v=_XBmxj2mKjM

12. *NBC News.* Trump, White House Coronavirus Task Force hold briefing. April 10, 2020; https://www.youtube.com/watch?v=Sk_VPy2CfCM.

13. *NBC News.* Trump and Coronavirus Task Force hold briefing at White House. April 2, 2020; https://www.youtube.com/watch?v=isosHlzEG0g.

14. *NBC News.* Trump and Coronavirus Task Force hold White House briefing. April 18, 2020; https://www.youtube.com/watch?v=Vf_waLOYm2k.

15. Luck AN, Preston SH, Elo IT, et al. The unequal burden of the COVID-19 pandemic: capturing racial/ethnic disparities in US cause-specific mortality. *SSM Popul Health.* 2022;17:101012.

16. Feldman JM, Bassett MT. Variation in COVID-19 mortality in the US by race and ethnicity and educational attainment. *JAMA Network Open.* 2021;4(11):e2135967.

17. Robert Wood Johnson Foundation, Harvard T.H. Chan School of Public Health. The public's perspective on the United States public health system. 2021; https://www.hsph.harvard.edu/wp-content/uploads/sites/94/2021/05/RWJF-Harvard-Report_FINAL-051321.pdf.

18. Marquez JR. A failure to communicate. *Georgia State University Research Magazine* 2020. https://news.gsu.edu/research-magazine/a-failure-to-communicate-covid-19-pandemic-public-health-messaging.

19. *NBC News.* Trump and Coronavirus Task Force hold White House briefing. April 17, 2020; https://www.youtube.com/watch?v=5QeZju3oBp0.

20. *NBC News.* Trump and Coronavirus Task Force brief from White House. March 26, 2020; https://www.youtube.com/watch?v=KIoGhR2JwLI.

21. Kinsella M, Fowler G, Boland J, et al. Trump administration abuses thwart US pandemic response. *The Brennan Center.* 2021; https://www.brennancenter.org/our-work/research-reports/trump-administration-abuses-thwart-us-pandemic-response.

22. Davis A. *Political Communication: A New Introduction for Crisis Times.* Cambridge: Polity; 2019.

23. Lloyd M, Friedland LA. *The Communication Crisis in America, and How to Fix It.* London: Palgrave MacMillan; 2016.

24. Garland R. *Government Communications and the Crisis of Trust: From Political Spin to Post-Truth.* London: Palgrave MacMillan; 2021.

25. Lilleker D, Coman IA, Gregor M, et al. *Political Communication and COVID-19: Governance and Rhetoric in Times of Crisis.* New York: Routledge; 2021.

26. Overton D, Ramkeesoon SA, Kirkpatrick K. Lessons from COVID-19 on executing communications and engagement at the community level during a health crisis. *National Academies of Science, Engineering, and Medicine.* 2021; https://www.nationalacademies.org/news/2021/12/lessons-from-covid-19-on-executing-communications-and-engagement-at-the-community-level-during-a-health-crisis.

27. Tofel RJ. How is America still this bad at talking about the pandemic? *The Atlantic. February* 2022; https://www.theatlantic.com/health/archive/2022/02/pandemic-communications-public-health/622044/.

28. Tyson A, Funk C. Increasing public criticism, confusion over COVID-19 response in U.S. *Pew Research Center.* 2022. https://www.pewresearch.org/science/2022/02/09/increasing-public-criticism-confusion-over-covid-19-response-in-u-s/

29. Hyland-Wood B, Gardner J, Leask J, et al. Toward effective government communication strategies in the era of COVID-19. *Humanit Soc Sci Commun.* 2021; 8(30).

30. Carter DP, May PJ. Making sense of the U.S. COVID-19 pandemic response: a policy regime perspective. *Admin Theory Prax.* 2020;42(2):265–277.

31. *Fox News.* President Trump goes one-on-one with Chris Wallace. July 19, 2020; https://www.youtube.com/watch?v=W6XdpDOH1JA.

32. Panzeri F, Di Paola S, Domaneschi F. Does the COVID-19 war metaphor influence reasoning? *PLoS ONE.* 2021;16(4):e0250651.

33. *PBS NewsHour.* Trump holds press conference on novel coronavirus. March 14, 2020; https://www.youtube.com/watch?v=TvHD1Jcx54w.

34. *NBC News.* White House COVID-19 Response Team briefing. January 26, 2022; https://www.youtube.com/watch?v=pPVInGkXGso.

35. *WCNC.* President Trump, White House coronavirus briefing. March 31, 2020; https://www.youtube.com/watch?v=PnA3SZnVJ_E&t=638s.

36. Larson HJ. *Stuck: How Vaccine Rumors Start and Why They Don't Go Away.* New York: Oxford University Press; 2020.

37. Burleigh N. *Virus, Vaccinations, the CDC, and the Hijacking of America's Response to the Pandemic.* New York: Seven Stories Press; 2021.

Chapter 5

1. Yeo AI, Green MN. *Living in an Age of Mistrust: An Interdisciplinary Study of Declining Trust and How to Get it Back*. New York: Routledge; 2017.
2. Thornton J. COVID-19: trust in government and other people linked with lower infection rate and higher vaccination uptake. *BMJ*. 2022;376:o292.
3. Liu J, Shahab Y, Hoque H. Government response measures and public trust during the COVID-19 pandemic: evidence from around the world. *Br J Manag*. 2022;33:571–602.
4. Dalton RJ. The social transformation of trust in government. *Int Rev Sociol*. 2005;15(1):133–154.
5. Hosking G. The decline of trust in government. In: Sasaki M, ed. *Trust in Contemporary Society*. Leiden: Brill; 2019, pp. 77–103.
6. Knight Commission on Trust, Media, and Democracy. Chapter 4: Why has trust in government and media declined? 2019; https://kf-site-production.s3.amazonaws.com/media_elements/files/000/000/283/original/Knight_Commission_Report_on_Trust_Media_and_Democracy_FINAL.pdf.
7. Doherty C, Kiley J, Asheer N, et al. Americans' view of government: decades of distrust, enduring support for its role. *Pew Research Center*. 2022. https://www.pewresearch.org/politics/2022/06/06/americans-views-of-government-decades-of-distrust-enduring-support-for-its-role/
8. OECD. Building trust to reinforce democracy: main findings from the 2021 OECD survey on drivers of trust in public institutions. 2022; https://www.oecd-ilibrary.org/sites/b407f99c-en/1/3/1/index.html?itemId=/content/publication/b407f99c-en&_csp_=c12e05718c887e57d9519eb8c987718b&itemIGO=oecd&itemContentType=book.
9. NPR, Kaiser Family Foundation, Harvard University Kennedy School of Government. Americans distrust government, but want it to do more. https://www.kff.org/wp-content/uploads/2013/01/americans-trust-government-but-want-it-to-do-more.pdf.
10. United Nations Department of Economic and Social Affairs. Trust in public institutions: trends and implications for economic security. 2021; https://www.un.org/development/desa/dspd/2021/07/trust-public-institutions/.
11. Halpin J, Nayak N, Teixeira R. Trust in government in the Trump era: a comprehensive study of U.S. public opinion on the federal government under the Trump administration. *Center for American Progress*. 2018; https://www.americanprogress.org/article/trust-government-trump-era/.
12. Niskanen Center. How the left and right undermined trust in government. 2021; https://www.niskanencenter.org/how-the-left-and-right-undermined-trust-in-government/.
13. Wilkerson I. *Caste: The Origins of Our Discontents*. New York: Random House; 2020.
14. Llewellyn S, Brookes S, Mahon A. *Trust and Confidence in Government and Public Services*. New York: Routledge; 2013.
15. Hitlin P, Shutava N. Trust in government: a close look at public perceptions of the federal government and its employees. *Partnership for Public Service*. 2022. https://ourpublicservice.org/wp-content/uploads/2022/03/Trust-in-Government.pdf
16. Case A, Deaton A. *Deaths of Despair and the Future of Capitalism*. Princeton, NJ: Princeton University Press; 2020.
17. Friedman J, Hansen H, Gone JP. Deaths of despair and Indigenous data genocide. *Lancet*. 2023;401(10379):874–876.
18. Babington C. Partisan views affect trust in government. *Pew Research Center*. 2021; https://www.pewtrusts.org/en/trust/archive/summer-2021/partisan-views-affect-trust-in-government.
19. McPhillips D. Survey: majority of Americans don't trust government with their health. *U.S. News & World Report*. March 26, 2020.
20. Geiersterfer-Black M, Niemi T, Neier L, et al. Trust in the U.S. government and its health agencies in the time of COVID-19. *Epidemiologia*. 2022;3(2):148–160.

21. Grandin G. *The End of the Myth: From the Frontier to the Border Wall in the Mind of America*. New York: Metropolitan Books; 2019.

22. Milbank D. *The Destructionists: The Twenty-Five Year Crack-Up of the Republic Party*. New York: Doubleday; 2022.

23. Hochschild AR. *Strangers in Their Own Land: Anger and Mourning on the American Right*. New York: The New Press; 2016.

24. Metzl JM. *Dying of Whiteness: How the Politics of Racial Resentment Is Killing America's Heartland*. New York: Basic Books; 2019.

25. Bollyky TJ, Hulland EN, Barber RM, et al. Pandemic preparedness and COVID-19: an exploratory analysis of infection and fatality rates, and contextual factors associated with preparedness in 177 countries, from Jan 1, 2020, to Sept 30, 2021. *Lancet*. 2022;399(10334):1489–1512.

26. Jordahl H. Inequality and trust. In: Svendsen GT, Svendsen GLH, eds. *Handbook of Social Capital* 2009. https://papers.ssrn.com/sol3/papers.cfm?abstract_id=1012786.

27. Sreedhar A, Gopal A. Behind low vaccination rates lurks a more profound social weakness. *New York Times. December 3,* 2021; https://www.nytimes.com/2021/12/03/opinion/vaccine-hesitancy-covid.html.

Chapter 6

1. Rainie L, Keeter S, Perrin A. Trust and distrust in America. *Pew Research Center*. 2019. https://www.pewresearch.org/politics/2019/07/22/trust-and-distrust-in-america/

2. Han Q, Zheng B, Cristea M, et al. Trust in government regarding COVID-19 and its associations with preventive health behaviour and prosocial behaviour during the pandemic: a cross-sectional and longitudinal study. *Psychol Med*. 2021;53(1):149–159. https://doi.org/ 10.1017/S0033291721001306.

3. Bobzien L. Income inequality and political trust: do fairness perceptions matter? *Soc Indic Res*. 2023;169:505–528.

4. Kawachi I, Kennedy BP, Lochner K, et al. Social capital, income inequality, and mortality. *Am J Public Health*. 1997;87(9):1491–1498.

5. Pickett KE, Wilkinson RG. Income inequality and health: a causal review. *Soc Sci Med*. 2015;128:316–326.

6. Daly M. *Killing the Competition: Economic Inequality and Homicide*. Piscataway, NJ: Transaction; 2016.

7. Filippi S, Schaffer M. Distrust in institutions: past, present, and future. *The Oxford Comment*. 2022; https://blog.oup.com/2022/09/distrust-in-institutions-past-present-and-future-podcast/.

8. Jones DR. Declining trust in Congress: effects of polarization and consequences for democracy. *Forum*. 2015;13(3):375–394.

9. Lee AHY. Social trust in polarized times: how perceptions of political polarization affect Americans' trust in each other. *Polit Behav*. 2022;44:1533–1554.

10. Fiorini S. Local news most trusted in keeping Americans informed about their communities. *Knight Foundation*. 2022; https://knightfoundation.org/articles/local-news-most-trusted-in-keeping-americans-informed-about-their-communities/.

11. Guess AM, Barberá P, Munzert S. The consequences of online partisan media. *PNAS*. 2021;118(14):e2013464118.

12. Bene M. Does context matter? a cross-country investigation of the effects of the media context on external and internal political efficacy. *Int J Comp Sociol*. 2020;61(4):264–286.

13. Van der Linden S. Misinformation: susceptibility, spread, and interventions to immunize the public. *Nat Med*. 2022;28:460–467.

14. Swire-Thompson B, Lazer D. Public health and online misinformation: challenges and recommendations. *Ann Rev Public Health*. 2020;41:433–451.

15. Lewandowsky S, Ecker EKH, Seifert CM, et al. Misinformation and its correction: continued influence and successful debiasing. *Psychol Sci Public Interest.* 2012;*13*(3):106–131.
16. Buczel M, Szyszka PD, Siwiak A, et al. Vaccination against misinformation: the inoculation technique reduces the continued influence effect. *PLoS ONE.* 2022;*17*(4):e0267463.
17. Pennycook G, Rand DG. Fighting misinformation on social media using crowdsourced judgments of news source quality. *PNAS.* 2019;*116*(7):2521–2526.
18. Edwards L, Stoilova M, Anstead N, et al. Rapid evidence assessment on online misinformation and media literacy final report. *Ofcom.* 2021.
19. Chan MS, Jones CR, Jamieson KH, et al. Debunking: a meta-analysis of the psychological efficacy of messages countering misinformation. *Psychol Sci.* 2017;*28*(11):1531–1546.
20. Gesser-Edelsburg A, Diamont A, Hijazi R, et al. Correcting health misinformation by health organizations during measles outbreaks: a controlled experiment. *PLoS ONE.* 2018;*13*(12):e0209505.
21. Bak-Coleman JB, Kennedy I, Wack M, et al. Combining interventions to reduce the spread of viral misinformation. *Nat Hum Behav.* 2022;*6*:1372–1380.
22. Roozenbeek J, Traberg CS, Van der Linden S. Technique-based inoculation against real-world misinformation. *R Soc Open Sci.* 2022;*9*:211719.
23. Van der Linden S, Roozenbeek J, Maertens R. How can psychological science help counter the spread of fake news? *Span J Psychol.* 2021;*24*:1–9.
24. Van der Linden S, Leiserowitz A, Rosenthal S, et al. Inoculating the public against misinformation about climate change. *Global Challenges.* 2017;*1*:1600008.
25. Sanalang A, Ophir Y, Cappella JN. The potential for narrative correctives to combat misinformation. *J Commun.* 2017;*69*:298–319.
26. Van der Linden S, Clarke CE, Maibach EW. Highlighting consensus among medical scientists increases public support for vaccines: evidence from a randomized experiment. *BMC Public Health.* 2015;*15*:1207.
27. Van der Meer T, Jin Y. Seeking formula for misinformation treatment in public health crises: the effects of corrective information type and source. *Health Commun.* 2020;*35*(5):560–575.
28. Ecker UKH, Lewandowsky S, Cook J, et al. The psychological drivers of misinformation belief and its resistance to correction. *Nat Rev Psychol.* 2022;*1*:13–29.
29. Gillory JJ, Geraci L. Correcting erroneous inferences in memory: the role of source credibility. *J Appl Res Mem Cogn.* 2013;*2*(4):201–209.
30. Ecker UKH, Antonio LM. Can you believe it? an investigation into the impact of retraction source credibility on the continued influence effect. *Mem Cogn.* 2021;*49*:631–644.
31. Amazeen M, Krishna A. Correcting vaccine misinformation: recognition and effects of source type on misinformation via perceived motivations and credibility. *Int J Commun.* 2023;*17*:560–582.
32. Aslett K, Guess AM, Bonneau R. News credibility labels have limited average effects on news diet quality and fail to reduce misperceptions. *Sci Adv.* 2022;*8*(18).
33. Stecula DA, Kuru O, Jamieson KH. How trust in experts and media use affect acceptance of common anti-vaccination claims. *HKS Misinformation Rev.* 2020;*1*(1):eabl3844.
34. OECD. Drivers of trust in public institutions in Norway. 2022; https://www.oecd.org/publications/drivers-of-trust-in-public-institutions-in-norway-81b01318-en.htm.
35. OECD. Drivers of trust in public institutions in Finland. 2021; https://www.oecd.org/fr/finlande/drivers-of-trust-in-public-institutions-in-finland-52600c9e-en.htm.
36. OECD. Understanding the drivers of trust in government institutions in Korea. 2018; https://www.oecd.org/korea/understanding-the-drivers-of-trust-in-government-institutions-in-korea-9789264308992-en.htm.
37. Carniel B. Misinformation superspreaders are thriving on Musk-owned Twitter. *Health Feedback.* 2023; https://healthfeedback.org/misinformation-superspreaders-thriving-on-musk-owned-twitter/?utm_source=Poynter+Institute&utm_campaign=95b546a7ae-factually1&utm_medium=email&utm_term=0_26742a15dc-95b546a7ae-393436616.

Conclusion

1. Wallis C. Information ecosystems: crafting and curating comprehensive systems for fact-finding and fact-checking. 2020; https://home.csulb.edu/~cwallis/170/text/Ecosystems3.pdf

2. Tokita CK, Guess AM, Tarnita CE. Polarized information ecosystems can reorganize social networks via information cascades. *PNAS*. 2021;*118*(50):e2102147118.

3. Anderson J, Rainie L. The future of truth and misinformation online. 2017. https://www.pewresearch.org/internet/2017/10/19/the-future-of-truth-and-misinformation-online/

4. Kleiner, K. How will we fix fake news? *University of Toronto Magazine*. 2020; https://magazine.utoronto.ca/research-ideas/culture-society/how-will-we-fix-fake-news.

5. Weeks BE. Emotions, partisanship, and misperceptions: how anger and anxiety moderate the effect of partisan bias on susceptibility to political misinformation. *J Commun*. 2015;*65*:699–719.

6. Salvi C, Iannello P, Cancer A, et al. Going viral: how fear, socio-cognitive polarization and problem-solving influence fake news detection and proliferation during the COVID-19 pandemic. *Front Commun*. 2021;*5*:562–588.

7. Barber SL, Lorenzoni L, Ong P. *Price Setting and Price Regulation in Health Care: Lessons for Advancing Universal Health Coverage*. Geneva: OECD; 2019.

8. Dubner SJ. How to fix the hot mess of U.S. healthcare. *Freakonomics*. 2021; https://freakonomics.com/podcast/how-to-fix-the-hot-mess-of-u-s-healthcare-ep-456/.

9. Bruhn WE, Rutkow L, Wang P. Prevalence and characteristics of Virginia hospitals suing patients and garnishing wages for unpaid medical bills. *JAMA*. 2019;*322*(7):691–692.

10. Keith K. Tracking the uninsured rate in 2019 and 2020. *Health Aff Forefront*. 2020.

11. National Center for Health Statistics. U.S. uninsured rate dropped 18% during pandemic. 2023; https://www.cdc.gov/nchs/pressroom/nchs_press_releases/2023/202305.htm.

12. Himmelstein DU, Lawless RM, Thorne D, et al. Medical bankruptcy: still common despite the Affordable Care Act. *Am J Public Health*. 2019;*109*(3):431–433.

13. Friedman W, Schleifer D. Taking the pulse: where Americans agree on improving health care. *Public Agenda/USA Today/Ipsos Hidden Common Ground Report*. 2020; https://publicagenda.org/wp-content/uploads/Taking-the-Pulse-Where-Americans-Agree-on-Improving-Health-Care_Final-2.pdf.

14. WHYY. Fixing the health care system: lessons from the pandemic. 2020; https://whyy.org/episodes/fixing-the-health-care-system-lessons-from-the-pandemic/.

15. National Center for Chronic Disease Prevention and Health Promotion. Our budget; https://www.cdc.gov/chronicdisease/programs-impact/budget/index.htm.

16. Simpson L. Fixing our fractured and failed health system. *AcademyHealth*. 2020; https://academyhealth.org/blog/2020-10/fixing our fractured and failed health-system.

17. Chernew ME, Cutler DM, Shah SA. Reducing health care spending: what tools can states leverage? *The Commonwealth Fund*. 2021; https://www.commonwealthfund.org/publications/fund-reports/2021/aug/reducing-health-care-spending-what-tools-can-states-leverage.

18. Whaley C, Frakt A. If patients don't use available health service pricing information, is transparency still important? *AMA J Ethics*. 2022;*24*(11):E1056–1062.

19. Butler SM. Achieving an equitable national health system for America. *The Brookings Institution*. 2020; https://www.brookings.edu/research/achieving-an-equitable-national-health-system-for-america/.

20. Kim S, Capasso A, Ali SH, et al. What predicts people's belief in COVID-19 misinformation? a retrospective study using a nationwide online survey among adults residing in the United States. *BMC Public Health*. 2022;*22*:2114.

21. Baumer-Mouradian SH, Hart RJ, Visotcky A, et al. Understanding influenza and SARS-CoV-2 vaccine hesitancy in racial and ethnic minority caregivers. *Vaccines*. 2022;*10*(11):1968.

22. Kim SJ, Schiffelbein JE, Imset I, et al. Countering antivax misinformation via social media: message-testing randomized experiment for human papillomavirus vaccination uptake. *J Med Internet Res*. 2022;*24*(11):e37559.
23. Pyenson B, Schulman M. There's nothing wrong with US health care that less money couldn't fix. Health Affairs Blog, December 6, 2019; https://www.healthaffairs.org/do/10.1377/forefront.20191205.766250/full/.
24. Engelmann J, Herrmann E. Chimpanzees trust their friends. *Curr Biol*. 2016;*6*(2):252–256.
25. Engelmann J, Herrmann E, Tomasello M. Chimpanzees trust conspecifics to engage in low-cost reciprocity. *Proc Biol Sci*. 2015;*282*(1801):20142803.
26. Ringer J, Chakrabarti M. Essential trust: trust in the animal kingdom. *WBUR*. 2022; https://www.wbur.org/onpoint/2022/11/28/essential-trust-trust-in-the-animal-kingdom-jane-goodall.
27. Liu F, Betts S. Between expectation and behavioral intent: a model of trust. *Proceedings of the Academy of Organizational Culture, Communications and Conflict*. 2003; https://www.researchgate.net/publication/305399492_Between_Expectation_and_Behavioral_Intent_A_Model_of_Trust.
28. Knack S, Zak PJ. Building trust: public policy, interpersonal trust, and economic development. *Supreme Court Economic Review*. 2003;*10*:91–107.
29. Zak, PJ, Knack S. Trust and growth. *SSRN*. 2002; https://ssrn.com/abstract=304639.
30. Willis J, Todorov A. First impressions: making up your mind after a 100-ms exposure to a face. *Psychol Sci*. 2006;*17*(7):592–598.
31. Chang J, Chakrabarti M. Essential trust: the brain science of trust. *WBUR*. 2022; https://www.wbur.org/onpoint/2022/11/29/essential-trust-how-our-brains-process-trust.
32. Sutherland P, Chakrabarti M. Essential trust: lessons from Brazil's trust crisis. *WBUR*. 2022; https://www.wbur.org/onpoint/2022/11/30/essential-trust-lessons-from-brazils-trust-crisis.
33. Sin SJ. Neighborhood disparities in access to information resources: measuring and mapping U.S. public libraries' funding and service landscapes. *Libr Inf Sci Res*. 2011;*33*(1):41–53.
34. Kelley MS, Su D, Britigan DH. Disparities in health information access: results of a county-wide survey and implications for health communication. *Health Commun*. 2016;*31*(5):575–582.
35. Yu J, Meng S. Impacts of the Internet on health inequality and healthcare access: a cross-country study. *Front Public Health*. 2022;*10*:935608.
36. Sloman S, Fernback P. *The Knowledge Illusion: Why We Never Think Alone*. New York: Riverhead Books; 2017.
37. Wehrman AM. *The Contagion of Liberty: The Politics of Smallpox in the American Revolution*. Baltimore, MD: Johns Hopkins University Press; 2022.
38. Kleinfeld R. Profound rebuilding needed to shore up U.S. democracy. *Carnegie Endowment for International Peace*. 2021; https://carnegieendowment.org/2021/01/07/profound-rebuilding-needed-to-shore-up-u.s.-democracy-pub-83575.
39. Ohio State Office of Academic Affairs. Restoring faith in American democracy. 2021.
40. Mounk Y. *The great experiment: why diverse democracies fall apart and how they can endure*. New York: Penguin Books; 2022.
41. Kalb J, Kuo D. Reassessing American democracy: the enduring challenge of racial exclusion. *Michigan Law Rev*. 2018;*117*:55–62. https://michiganlawreview.org/reassessing-american-democracy-the-enduring-challenge-of-racial-exclusion/.
42. Manthorpe J. *Restoring democracy in the age of populists and pestilence*. Toronto: Cormorant Books; 2020.
43. Arendt H. *The Origins of Totalitarianism*. San Diego: Harcourt; 1973.
44. Renström EA, Bäck H, Knapton HM. Exploring a pathway to radicalization: the effects of social exclusion and rejection sensitivity. *Group Process Intergr Relat*. 2020;*23*(8):1204–1229.

45. Brown RA, Helmus TC, Ramchand R, et al. *What Do Former Extremists and Their Families Say About Radicalization and Deradicalization in America?* Santa Monica, CA: RAND; 2021.

46. Langenkamp A, Bientsman S. Populism and layers of social belonging: support of populist parties in Europe. *Polit Psychol.* 2022;*43*(5):931–949.

Further Reading

This book covers a lot of ground from several different disciplines. There were a lot of sources consulted that did not make it into the notes but are still incredibly useful if readers are interested in delving deeper. Here is a suggested list for further reading, broken out by themes discussed in this book.

The American Healthcare System

Makary M. *The Price We Pay: What Broke American Health Care—and How to Fix It.* London: Bloomsbury; 2019.

Messac L. *Your Money or Your Life: Debt Collection in American Medicine.* Oxford: Oxford University Press; 2023.

Crisis Communications and Pandemic Preparedness

Alexander M, Unruh L, Koval A, et al. United States response to the COVID-19 pandemic, January–November 2020. *Health Econ Policy Law.* 2021;17(1):62–75.

Altman D. Understanding the US failure on coronavirus. *BMJ.* 2020;370:m3417.

Gontariuk M, Krafft T, Rehbock C, et al. The European Union and public health emergencies: expert opinions on the management of the first wave of the COVID-19 pandemic and suggestions for future emergencies. *Front Public Health.* 2021;9:698995.

Hanage WP, Testa C, Chen JT, et al. COVID-19: US federal accountability for entry, spread, and inequities—lessons for the future. *Eur J Epidemiol.* 2020;35:995–1006.

Hatcher, W. A failure of political communication not a failure of bureaucracy: the danger of presidential misinformation during the COVID-19 pandemic. *Am Rev Public Admin.* 2020;50(6–7):614–620.

Hyland-Wood B, Gardner J, Leask J, et al. Toward effective government communication strategies in the era of COVID-19. *Humanit Soc Sci Commun.* 2021;8:30.

Kim DKD, Kreps GL. An analysis of government communication in the United States during the COVID-19 pandemic: recommendations for effective government health risk communication. *World Med Health Policy.* 2020;12(4):398–412.

Lilleker D, Coman IA, Gregor M, et al., eds. *Political Communication and COVID-19: Governance and Rhetoric in Times of Crisis.* Abingdon: Routledge; 2021.

Merkley E, Loewen PJ. Anti-intellectualism and the mass public's response to the COVID-19 pandemic. *Nat Hum Behav.* 2021;5:706–721.

Nuzzo JB, Bell JA, Cameron EE. Suboptimal US response to COVID-19 despite robust capabilities and resources. *JAMA.* 2020;324(14):1391–1392.

Sauer MA, Truelove S, Gerste AK, et al. A failure to communicate? how public messaging has strained the COVID-19 response in the United States. *Health Secur.* 2021;19(1):65–74.

Sell TK, Hosangadi D, Trotochaud M. Misinformation and the US Ebola communication crisis: analyzing the veracity and content of social media messages related to a fear-inducing infectious disease outbreak. *BMC Public Health.* 2020;20:550.

The Nature and Future of Democracy

Applebaum A. *Twilight of Democracy: The Seductive Lure of Authoritarianism.* New York: Doubleday; 2020.

Manthorpe J. *Restoring Democracy in an Age of Populists and Pestilence*. Toronto: Cormorant Books; 2021.

Nelson A. *Shadow Network: Media, Money, and the Secret Hub of the Radical Right*. London: Bloomsbury; 2021.

Pitcavage M. *Surveying the Landscape of the American Far Right*. Washington, DC: GW Program on Extremism; 2019.

Rachman G. *Age of the Strongman: How the Cult of the Leader Threatens Democracy Around the World*. New York: Random House; 2021.

Runciman D. *The Confidence Trap: A History of Democracy From World War I to the Present*. Princeton, NJ: Princeton University Press; 2015.

Racism in Medicine and the Healthcare System

Baumer-Mauradian SH, Hart RJ, Visotcky A, et al. Understanding influenza and SARS- CoV-2 vaccine hesitancy in racial and ethnic minority caregivers. *Vaccines*. 2022;10(11):1968.

Jimenez ME, Rivera-Núñes Z, Crabtree BF, et al. Black and Latinx community perspectives on COVID-19 mitigation behaviors, testing, and vaccines. *JAMA Network Open*. 2021;4(7):e2117074.

Opel DJ, Lo B, Peek ME. Addressing mistrust about COVID-19 vaccines among people of color. *Ann Intern Med*. 2021.

Villarosa, Linda. *Under the Skin: The Hidden Toll of Racism on American Lives and on the Health of Our Nation*. New York: Random House; 2022.

Wells L, Gowda A. A legacy of mistrust: African Americans and the US healthcare system. *Proceed UCLA Health*. 2020;24.

Conspiracy Theories

Ahmed W, Segui F, Vidal-Alaball J, et al. COVID-19 and the "film your hospital" conspiracy theory: social network analysis of Twitter data. *J Med Internet Res*. 2020;22(10):e22374.

Douglas KM. Covid-19 conspiracy theories. *Group Process Intergr Relat*. 2021;24(2):27–175.

Freeman D, Waite F, Rosebrock L, et al. Coronavirus conspiracy beliefs, mistrust, and compliance with government guidelines in England. *Psychol Med*. 2022;52:251–265.

Gerts D, Shelley CD, Parikh N, et al. "Thought I'd share first" and other conspiracy theory tweets from the COVID-19 infodemic: exploratory study. *JMIR Public Health Surveill*. 2021;7(4):e26527.

Grimes DR. Medical disinformation and the unviable nature of COVID-19 conspiracy theories. *PLoS ONE*. 2021;16(3):e0245900.

Lahrach Y, Furnham A. Are modern health worries associated with medical conspiracy theories? *J Psychosom Res*. 2017;99:89–94.

Miller BL. Science denial and COVID conspiracy theories: potential neurological mechanisms and possible responses. *JAMA*. 2020;324(22):2255–2256.

Romer D, Jamieson KH. Conspiracy theories as barriers to controlling the spread of COVID-19 in the U.S. *Soc Sci Med*. 2020;263:113356.

Sauermilch D. HIV Conspiracy theory belief or institutional mistrust? a call for disentangling key concepts. *AIDS Res Human Retrovir*. 2020;36(3):171–172.

Vaccine Hesitancy

Cascini F, Pantovic A, Al-Ajilouni Y, et al. Social media and attitudes towards a COVID-19 vaccination: a systematic review of the literature. *EClinicalMed*. 2022;48:101454.

Hotez P. *Preventing the Next Pandemic: Vaccine Diplomacy in a Time of Anti-Science*. Baltimore, MD: Johns Hopkins University Press; 2021.

Jones DL, Salazar AS, Rodriguez VJ, et al. Severe acute respiratory syndrome coronavirus 2: vaccine hesitancy among underrepresented racial and ethnic groups with HIV in Miami, Florida. *Open Forum Infect Dis*. 2021;26;8(6):ofab154.

Joshi A, Kaur M, Kaur R, et al. Predictors of COVID-19 vaccine acceptance, intention, and hesitancy: a scoping review. *Front Public Health*. 2021;13;9:698111.
Kricorian K, Civen R, Equils O. COVID-19 vaccine hesitancy: misinformation and perceptions of vaccine safety. *Hum Vaccin Immunother*. 2022;18(1):1950504.

Trust, Distrust, and Misinformation

Cheung ATM, Parent B. Mistrust and inconsistency during COVID-19: considerations for resource allocation guidelines that prioritise healthcare workers. *J Med Ethics*. 2021;47:73–77.
Garland R. *Government Communications and the Crisis of Trust: From Political Spin to Post-Truth*. London: Palgrave Macmillan; 2021.
Han Q, Zheng B, Cristea M. Trust in government regarding COVID-19 and its associations with preventive health behaviour and prosocial behaviour during the pandemic: a cross-sectional and longitudinal study. *Psychol Med*. 2023;53(1):149–159.
Mabillard V. Trust in government: assessing the impact of exposure to information in a local context. *Int J Public Admin*. 2022;45(9):687–696.
Pilgrim D, Vassilev I. *Examining Trust in Healthcare: A Multidisciplinary Perspective*. London: Red Globe Press; 2010.
Reierson J, Roll K, Williams JD. Trust: a double-edged sword in combating the COVID-19 pandemic? *Front Commun*. 2022;7:822302.
Saltz E, Barari S, Liebowicz C. Misinformation interventions are common, divisive, and poorly understood. *HKS Misinformation Rev*. 2021;2(5):1–24.
Shore DA, ed. *The Trust Crisis in Healthcare*. Oxford: Oxford University Press; 2006.
Soveri A, Karlsson LC, Antfok J. Unwillingness to engage in behaviors that protect against COVID-19: the role of conspiracy beliefs, trust, and endorsement of complementary and alternative medicine. *BMC Public Health*. 2021;21:684.
Wang Y, McKee M, Torbica A. systematic literature review on the spread of health-related misinformation on social media. *Soc Sci Med*. 2019;240:112552.
Wolfensberger M, Wrigley A. *Trust in Medicine: Its Nature, Justification, Significance, and Decline*. Cambridge: Cambridge University Press; 2019.
Yang Z, Luo X, Jia H. Is it all a conspiracy? conspiracy theories and people's attitude to COVID-19 vaccination. *Vaccines*. 2021;9:1051.
Zuckerman E. *Mistrust: Why Losing Faith in Institutions Provides the Tools to Transform Them*. New York: W.W. Norton; 2021.

Index

For the benefit of digital users, indexed terms that span two pages (e.g., 52–53) may, on occasion, appear on only one of those pages.